Introduction to the Anatomy and Physiology of Children

Fully updated, this new edition provides an introduction to normal, healthy physical development for all professionals who specialise in working with children. The author, an experienced nurse teacher, guides the reader through the key changes in body systems and functions from embryo to birth through childhood and adolescence.

Chapter 1 sets the scene for physical needs in child development, such as the need to be warm and safe. Chapters 2 to 9 cover the body systems:

- skeletal
- nervous
- cardiovascular
- respiratory
- renal
- digestive
- reproductive
- immune.

The embryology and physiological function at birth is explored in each chapter before the text moves on through the many changes over the next decade to puberty and the arrival at adult functioning. A new final chapter provides a holistic account of children's development, body and mind. Each chapter is illustrated with line drawings and tables, and ends with scenarios which illustrate how knowledge supports good practice in a real-life situation, and a quiz to consolidate learning.

Concise and clearly written, this introductory text will be essential reading for all those working with children and families in the health and social care sector who must be aware of Every Child Matters and new national service framework government directives to ensure children enjoy a safe and healthy childhood.

Janet MacGregor was the Faculty of Health and Social Care Director of Knowledge Transfer and Foundation Degrees at Canterbury Christ Church University. She is now Principal of the College of Nursing at Fatima Memorial System, Lahore, Pakistan.

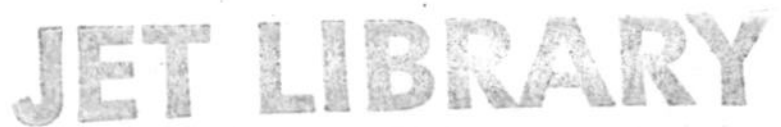

Dedication

This book is dedicated to my students and the children we care for.

I am particularly grateful to six 'little people', whom I have studied closely in compiling this book:

Morgan
George
Annabel
Hamish
Louise
Cameron

May these reflections on your individual development help those who are interested in other children's physical development to understand all children's needs and thus provide the optimum environment for them to achieve their unique genetic potential.

Thank you.

Introduction to the Anatomy and Physiology of Children

A guide for students of nursing, child care and health

Second edition

Janet MacGregor

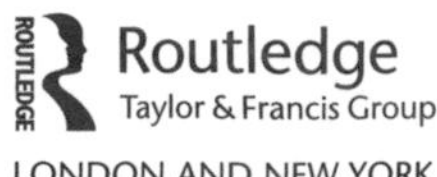
Routledge
Taylor & Francis Group
LONDON AND NEW YORK

First published 2000

This edition published 2008
by Routledge
2 Park Square, Milton Park,
Abingdon, Oxon OX14 4RN

Simultaneously published in the USA and Canada
by Routledge
270 Madison Ave, New York, NY 10016

Routledge is an imprint of the Taylor & Francis Group, an informa business

Typeset in Janson and Futura by
Florence Production Ltd, Stoodleigh, Devon
Printed and bound in Great Britain by
TJ International Ltd, Padstow, Cornwall

British Library Cataloguing in Publication Data
A catalogue record for this book is available from the British Library

Library of Congress Cataloging in Publication Data

MacGregor, Janet, 1943–
Introduction to the anatomy and physiology of children: a guide for students of nursing, child care, and health/
Janet MacGregor. – 2nd ed.
p.cm.
Includes bibliographical references and index
1. Children–Physiology. 2. Human anatomy. 3. Child development.
I. Title.
RJ125.M23 2008
612′.0083–dc22 2007038191

ISBN10: 0–415–44623–6 (hbk)
ISBN10: 0–415–44624–4 (pbk)
ISBN10: 0–203–92931–4 (ebk)

ISBN13: 978–0–415–44623–5 (hbk)
ISBN13: 978–0–415–44624–2 (pbk)
ISBN13: 978–0–203–92931–5 (ebk)

Contents

Illustrations

Figures

Tables

Preface

This book is not a comprehensive guide to children's physical development, but an introduction to some selected topics commonly discussed with a variety of students working in child health contexts, and for parents who wish to provide the optimum environment for their offspring to flourish.

There is a wide range of 'normal' at any age, no more so than in the period before adult attributes are attained. However, there are physical milestones that all children reach in a definite sequence, and these milestones are universal. Most parents note the age their baby rolls and sits; most teachers know which skills their pupils should be able to perform; most health professionals know the parameters of their small charges' vital signs. The content of this book is aimed at all those who are responsible for the care of children, and will first set the scene for physical development to take place.

In September 2004, the government of England published directives for all those who have responsibilities for children (Every Child Matters), which proposed a range of reforms to ensure children's health and security were secured. Five principles underpin this government directive, the first being for the child to be physically and mentally healthy. A common core of knowledge was advised for all those who work with children and families. This text addresses the need to understand healthy physical growth and then offers a chance to understand the damage to health when children smoke, become pregnant in their teenage years or eat abnormally, for example.

This text begins with two development theories which have been chosen to present the nature–nurture effect on physical change. Some selected topics are then addressed, such as healthy environments and health promotion issues, which should facilitate children's optimal growth. The succeeding chapters then investigate the body systems in more detail, where it is hoped the reader will be stimulated to take his or her own interest further and research some of the topics more fully. The final chapter takes the reader back from the physical to the psychological, and thus completes the circle, where a healthy body is intricately entwined with a happy child.

Chapter 1

Child physical needs

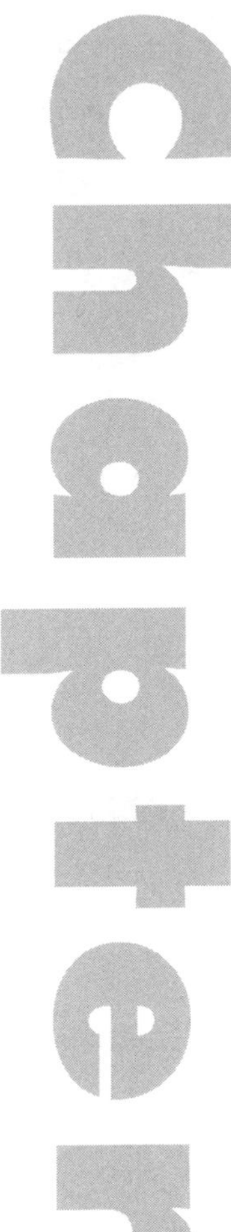

- Child development theories
- The nature–nurture debate
- Genetic inheritance
- A healthy environment
- The need for protective care
- The need for food
- The need for temperature control
- The need for activity, rest and sleep

THE PHYSICAL DEVELOPMENT of children is part of their whole development and therefore must be seen in the context of the social, emotional and intellectual changes that occur through childhood. Child development theories reflect the philosophies of their various authors, but as the subject is so complex, they have often been formulated from a particular stance. For this discussion, two theories have been selected to support the genetic and environmental effects on physical change. Inherited influences can be both subtle and obvious, as can the more long-term effects of environment. The effects of both interact over many years from conception to old age; they are instrumental in changing the child as it physically grows and matures.

Child development theories

Bee and Boyd (2007) suggest that there are three fundamental child development concepts that need to be understood:

- the way in which children are the same and different;
- the internal and external influences on these changes;
- whether changes are quantitative or qualitative in nature.

To this end, there are two groups of theories on development that are helpful in understanding the changes that occur in the 'physical' child, and reflect the internal and external nature of the influences for change. These are the biological theories and the learning theories.

Biological theories are based on common patterns of development and the unique individual behavioural tendencies that are partially programmed by genetic inheritance. The development of sitting, for example, occurs as the maturation of systems allows this skill to occur. There is some acknowledgement that the child must be in an environment that facilitates this, and that s/he has the inclination to do so.

The biological changes are both quantitative and qualitative in nature; children can be 'aged' by the degree of ossification of their skeletal system. However, their genetic inheritance, the degree of activity they have experienced and their usual diet will ensure children will all be slightly different. It is with this biological philosophy that the succeeding chapters will explore the physical changes that occur in childhood.

The second group of theories comprises the learning theories, which propose that only reflexes are inherited and that all subsequent behavioural changes are learnt. For such theorists the environmental influence is most important, together with the process within that of learning. The 'learnt' behaviour that takes place can only be inferred from observing the 'changed' behaviour. It is a 'learnt' behaviour that must be relatively permanent and which results from past experience (Gross 2005). These 'learnt' behaviours then become cumulative in nature, and require memory to allow them to develop. They are qualitative in nature – the children can be seen to perform a skill more successfully as they increase in maturity and experience. Children learning to skip show this qualitative development; at first they cannot coordinate the rope with their feet, but with practise they soon develop sophisticated movements as they work with the rope. A 'learnt' behaviour can also arise from a conditional response, such as the child being praised for eating lunch. This is called the law of effect, where there is a pleasurable experience in performing a task that perhaps is not initiated by the child. Much behavioural therapy uses this technique when the temper tantrum is ignored but the acceptable response rewarded. An alternative learning theory is that of watching rather than doing; the learnt behaviour developing through an interpersonal situation. Here the child will watch a role model and see the consequence of this model's actions. Young children watch older children using the toilet and being praised for this action, so they will mimic their behaviour. They also see older children scream and shout to get their own way, and copy this! If children value the result of an action they will use the behaviour themselves, sometimes to their detriment, such as when the adolescent seeks affection from the peer group through antisocial activity.

The nature–nurture debate

The nature–nurture debate reflects the biological and learning theories discussed above. Inherited and environmental factors are both shown to play an important role in ensuring that the child will develop into a unique individual, but these are complex interactions on individuals with different characteristics. Werner and Smith (2001) showed how children growing up together in a poor Hawaiian environment had both positive and negative outcomes as adults due to inherent characteristics that they termed 'vulnerable' or 'resilient'. A recent UNICEF – the United Nations Children's Fund – survey of the rich countries of the world in 2007, used forty indicators of countries' nurturing environment and commitment to child welfare; themes used were of material wellbeing, family and peer relationships, health and safety, behaviour and risks, educational wellbeing and subjective wellbeing. Sadly, the UK was found to be wanting in five of the six categories of optimal facilities for healthy child development (UNICEF 2007).

Adult height is achieved through the interaction of the inherited potential from both parents and the child growing in an optimum environment, where they receive adequate nutrition and are free from disease. This complex interaction between inheritance and the need for supportive environment may be seen in populations where food is scarce and ethnic unrest ongoing. Ethnic groups who change their diet and lifestyle, and perhaps marry into the indigenous race when settling into a new country, may see their children's physical growth and maturation change over future generations (McQuaid *et al.* 1996). However, Kmietowicz (2006) suggests that children will develop within the same range of height and weight anywhere in the world given healthy growth conditions and advises that the World Health Organisation (WHO) growth charts can now be used globally (www.who.int/childgrowth/en/).

Genetic inheritance

Inherited characteristics are transmitted from one generation to the next in a random way, and they strongly affect the end result of growth and the progress towards it. There is a high correlation of a child and its parent regarding height, weight, shape and form of features, body build and skin colour. Many dimensions of personality, such as temperament, also seem to be inherited. Inherited potential is decided at conception as the genes from both father and mother combine to form the new unique individual, according to the principle of independent assortment at meiosis (Thibodeau and Patton 2007).

Early research established that some genes were dominant to others and held the more likely characteristics to be expressed, such as hair and eye colour. Recessive genes, those that were 'hidden' by the dominant genes, provide the 'throwback' phenomenon produced when both parents carry the recessive characteristic. However, many human traits are controlled by multiple alleles (see below), or polygenes, and thus are not perfect predictions (Marieb and Hoehn 2007). Skin colour is a polygene controlled by three separately inherited genes each in two allelic forms – *Aa*, *Bb* and *Cc*. Remember that chromosomes are paired for characteristics thus genes are paired and these are called alleles. *ABC* confers dark skin pigment; *abc* confers pale skin tone, and the effects are additive (see Figure 1.1).

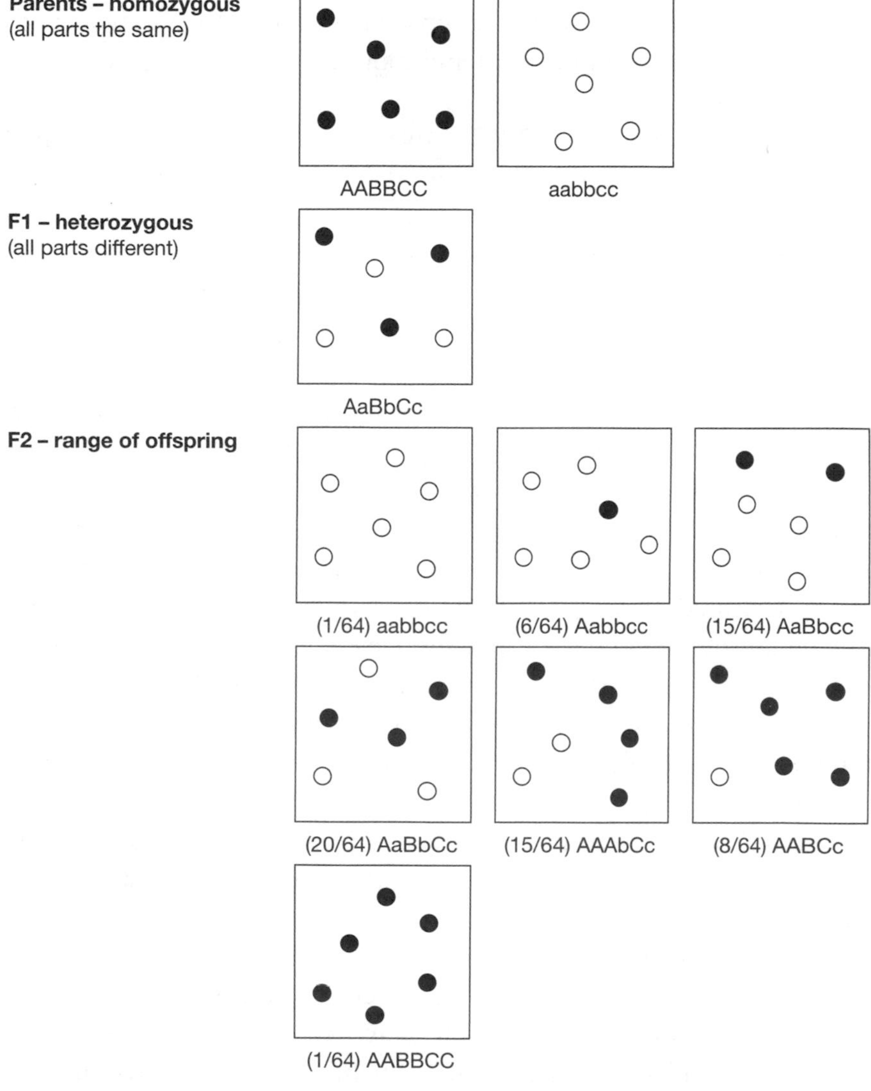

Figure 1.1 Skin colour inheritance

Thus *AABBCC* genetic inheritance gives very dark skin and *aabbcc* gives very pale skin. The inheritance pattern for skin colour leads to a broad range of offspring. It is also now commonly believed that many genes are not individually expressed, but interact or link in inherited characteristics that produce many of an individual's features. The unusual colouring of red hair and green eyes, or the unexpected stature of a very small son or daughter, may be examples of this phenomenon. Genetically inherited characteristics can also be seen in the distinct racial groups. Afro-Caribbean children develop their muscular skeletal systems in advance of white or Chinese children, regardless of their diet or environment. Black babies hold their heads up well, and may sit and stand earlier than those of other racial groups.

Thibodeau and Patten (2007) explain how the Human Genome, first described in 2003, consists of forty-six individual nuclear chromosomes and one mitochromal chromosome made of DNA and is subdivided into 20,000 to 25,000 genes. Chromosomes are also of different sizes. Chromosome 1 has 3,000 genes and the Y chromosome, required for male characteristics, has only 200. This explains how the important proteins making genes are only 2 per cent of the total DNA material found in the nucleus of every body cell and that the genetic code consists of much 'packing' nucleic material with no known function of characteristic expression. Apart from the basic sequencing of the genome, and the plan to study human genetic variation and human susceptibility to disease, the Human Genome Project also sequenced the genomes of other important organisms, including the mouse, yeast, fruit fly, Japanese puffer fish and roundworm. They found the same number of genes in the rat and the mouse as in the human sequence and that the human sequence was only one and a half times the number found in the nuclei of the fruit fly cells.

New treatments using genetic engineering are already today helping infertile couples to conceive their children using artificially stimulated oogenesis, donated eggs and sperms, and 'wombs for rent'. The cloning of animals has been successful, and the manufacture of medications which replicate the genetic patterning of the natural product, such as insulin, is widely practised. Genetic scientists can predict sex and some physical abnormalities; the construction of a human child is not a dream.

A healthy environment

Physical health in children's early years is of paramount importance; they must be given the best possible chance of a healthy future. As they grow and change, so their health needs change for them to achieve their genetic potential. Many factors influence their physical health before and after birth. Children's views about their health also change as they experience the world and adapt and refine their purpose in life. London *et al.* (2006) offer a WHO (2001) definition of health as a state of complete physical, mental and social wellbeing and not merely the absence of disease and infirmity. It is viewed as dynamic, changing and unfolding: it is the realisation of a state of actualisation or potential (Pender *et al.* 2002). This developmental approach to health promotion for children is most appropriate, as it parallels the development of cognitive processes. Thus, children of six years will see health in a 'concrete' way, enabling them to do what they want to do – play outside and go to school. The teenager, however, will find the task of defining health more difficult and probe the questioner for context, seeing health as something more 'abstract' that involves both body and mind.

Health projects in cities aimed at making the environment more friendly to children, such as the Healthy Cities Project, initiated by WHO, have now been extended to the worldwide Healthy Cities Movement. In 2001, Takano and Nakamura showed how the nine determinants of a health city had a high level of correlation to the health index of the population. One of its targets relates to health-promoting physical and social environments, concentrating professional help into empowering populations to develop skills that allow them to make healthy choices for living (Twinn *et al.* 1998). All children need safe areas for physical play, away from pollution, noise and traffic, and they need to be encouraged to be physically active in recreations they enjoy (see Chapters 2–4 on the skeletal, muscular and cardiovascular systems).

The following topics for health promotion are offered as important to optimal physical development:

- the need for protective care;
- the need for food;
- the need for temperature control;
- the need for activity and rest.

The need for protective care

Children depend not only on their immediate carers for protection but on the policies of the state to create a safe environment in which they can thrive. Hall and Elliman (2003) stressed the importance of promoting child health in the community, and one of their key recommendations was for accident prevention measures. All body systems require freedom from the stresses of pain, anxiety and medical interventions, which are often part of the accident and illness experience, to develop their full potential. It is when children experience either visible or invisible (biological) harm that the development of their physical self is seen to suffer (see the section on stress in the discussion of the immune system in Chapter 9).

Protection from visible risks – accidental and non-accidental injury

Accidental injury

Accidents are the single most reported cause of death in children between the ages of one and fifteen years; children are seen as adventurous, unpredictable and fun-seeking. However, those minor accidents that happen in the home are rarely reported and perhaps are part of growing up. Children can be clumsy, impetuous and curious, and their carers can be ignorant of their needs and lax in supervision. Families may live in poverty and the children disadvantaged: Polnay (2002) describes the impact of poverty as both physical and/or behavioural. Roberts *et al.* (1998) reported the increasing injury death rate gradients for children under the age of fifteen years in UK social class V from 1991 to 1995, with the risks highest for fire and homicide, underscoring the strong relationship between violence and poverty. However, the overall death rates for children in the UK are decreasing and were lower than in the USA and Australia in 1995, where teenage death due to use of firearms for homicide or suicide were rising (Department of Health 1999). They suggest that this may be, in part, due to safer home and local environments, advances in medical science and easy access to health care. However, constant minor injuries and their frequent association with infections that do not kill may result in children expending their energy for tissue repair rather than for growth.

The infant is at risk of falling due to the innate reflexes propelling the child forward, for example, from the baby chair if not strapped in. Babies soon start to roll, and may roll from a changing mat to the floor. At six months, small objects may be ingested or inhaled as the baby grasps and investigates with its mouth. When crawling is achieved, the child will not know that interesting objects on the floor are dangerous to explore with its mouth or to eat. However, the biggest threat to this age, as identified in a 1995 survey (see below), was suffocation due to inhalation or ingestion of foreign bodies (Roberts *et al.* 1998).

Young school-aged children are only beginning to understand causal relationships and to think about the effects of their actions. They have improving muscle coordination and want to practise and perfect their physical skills. Cycling is a favourite activity for this age group, but in the excitement of the chase they may forget to watch for cars that share the public domain. They are increasingly exposed to more and various environments, and are easily distracted from a safe course by things that are seen as more interesting. The 1995 survey (Twinn *et al.* 1998) found pedestrian accidents and road traffic accidents the major cause of their injury and unintentional death.

Teenagers have often progressed to activities involving motorbikes and alcohol, which may frequently lead to involvement in fights. Children of this age group have a need to establish themselves as independent and responsible for their own actions, and this command over their own lives may lead them to feel indestructible. They may not consider the consequences of their actions if peer group pressure is strong: teenage pregnancy, sexually transmitted disease and mental disorders are rising and poverty is still apparent in these young people's lives (Viner and Booy 2005). They also participate in more sporting activities, and are thus more exposed to physical injury (Wong *et al.* 2003). Viner and Booy (2005) and Carnidge *et al.* (2003) show how social problems, road traffic accidents and drug/alcohol overdose are increasingly the cause of teenage death, either accidentally or when intending suicide.

Non-accidental injury

Child abuse is often the result of family stress and a need for parenting skills, and can be compounded by children frightened to ask for help.

Cawson *et al.* (2000), in their study for the National Society for the Prevention of Cruelty to Children (NSPCC), defined physical, sexual and emotional abuse collectively as maltreatment which resulted in harm in varying degrees and over differing time spans. Jose (2005) argues that poverty is society's neglect and also a form of child abuse. The DH (2003), in Lord Laming's inquiry into the death of a child maltreated by her aunt, stated that protecting children from harm is everyone's business and the responsibility of all those who care for them individually. However, abuse of children is context dependent, a socially defined construct that is the product of time and culture (Corby 2006): in some countries child labour, which is legally controlled in the UK, may be seen as useful to the family survival in under developed economies where children at work are ensured food to eat and are valued members of the extended family. Few single influences on development however, including severe abuse, have inevitable future consequences for the child. It is the sum and direction of many positive and negative influences that will have a bearing on the eventual outcome of any child's adjustment in adult life. One of the common indicators of any abuse is that the child will physically fail to thrive (see Chapter 10).

Behavioural expressions, such as the frozen watchfulness in the toddler, overfriendliness in the school-aged child and the teenager who looks for a confidante, groomed by an abuser, should alert the professional carer to a child needing protection (Trigge and Mohammed 2006). The Common Assessment Framework includes these indicators (DH 2006).

For a child to develop, he or she needs a secure attachment from which to explore the world and to return to when anxious or distressed (Barker and Hodes 2004). Bowlby (2000) stresses the important long-term effect of good/bad attachment experience on the physical, social and emotional self as the child 'unfolds' over time.

The child needs a secure attachment to:

- attain his or her full intellectual potential;
- sort out what he or she perceives;
- think logically;
- develop a conscience;
- become self-reliant;
- cope with stress and frustration;
- handle fear and worry;

- develop future relationships;
- handle jealousy.

Bee and Boyd (2007) explain how children's social cognition develops in certain directions:

- From outer to inner characteristic: where a young child pays attention to the surface of things, what things look like; the older child looks for principles, for causes.
- From observation to inference: the young child bases their conclusions on what they can see or feel; the older child will make inferences about what ought to be or might be.
- From definite to qualified: the young child's rules are fixed whereas the older child will 'bend' the rules to suit different contexts.
- From observer's view to general rule: the child becomes less egocentric and is able to use experience to construct a view more applicable to everyone.

There appears to be a lack of agreement on the basic rights of children among professionals who aim to protect them from harm. The Children Act (2004), in certain circumstances, allows for the child's wishes to be taken into consideration in any action involving them, but the family with whom they live may be permitted to have parental responsibility for decision-making, as children are considered to be physically weak, immature and powerless (Barker and Hodes 2004). This has resulted in professionals needing to intervene in normal family functions in order to protect the child (DfES 2006). Child protection is now perceived as distinct from child care, and the product of a relationship between the state, the family and the child to support the child's human rights (www.everychildmatters.gov.uk/socialcare/safeguarding).

Protection from invisible (biological) risk – immunisation

Immunisation programmes are available for all children in the UK free of charge. The schedule at present offers protection against:

- diphtheria, tetanus, pertussus, polio haemophilus (DTaP/IPV/Hib) and pneumococcus at two months;
- DTaP/IPV/Hib with meningitis C (MenC) at three months;
- DTaP/IPV/Hib with pneumococcus protection at four months;
- Hib and meningitis C at twelve months;
- measles, mumps and rubella with pneumococcus at thirteen months;
- boosters for MMR/DTaP/IPV vaccinations at three to five years and boosters for dT/IPV at thirteen to eighteen years.

(Chief Medical Officer 2006, Diggle 2006, Glasper *et al.* 2007, regular update at www.immunisation.nhs.uk)

Today, these diseases are rarely seen; thus parents have become more concerned with the side-effects of the vaccines on healthy children than with the effects of the infections themselves. However, Samad (2006) noted that herd protection was high in the UK and that out of 18,488 families surveyed in 2000–2002, 3.3 per cent were partially immunised and only 1.1 per cent were unimmunised in the population. The debate surrounding the measles, mumps and rubella (MMR) injections suggests, perhaps, that a more enlightened partnership with parents is required by the government and health professionals of the day. The vaccination controversies move on: Coombes (2007) reports on the prevention of the cervical cancer initiative where ten-year-old girls can be offered five years of protection from incubating the papillomavirus, a viral infection transmitted during sexual intercourse. Parents are unhappy with the sexual health knowledge needed to advise this age group. Bellaby (2003) suggests that concordance is the aim if compliance is to fall into place; many more children are killed or maimed by road traffic accidents than by vaccination and the relative risks have to be communicated effectively by the professionals for parent attitudes in a modern democracy to change.

The need for food

Dietary habits have shown some healthy trends in the past thirty years. Less red meat, butter, cake and biscuits are consumed, and more poultry, fresh fruit and brown bread eaten. A healthy diet should be based on a wide variety of foods, and for children under five years, with emphasis on those foods of high nutrient density rather than those providing energy only (Robinson 2006, Taylor *et al.* 2004). This balanced diet can be achieved by selecting items from four food groups each day (Costain 2007 and MacNair 2007). Three can be taken from lean meat, fish, poultry, game, eggs, pulses and nuts; three from milk, cheese and yoghurt; four from bread, rice, pasta, breakfast cereal and potatoes; four from vegetables and fruit. Chan (1995) describes the Chinese custom of balancing the diet with reference to hot (Yang) and cold (Yin) foods, in order to ensure continuing health and to restore health after illness.

Malnutrition and the subsequent detrimental effect on physical development can result from lack of food, the wrong food and too much food. The effect of diet starts in the womb, the foetus relies on the mother to provide all the necessary nutrients for growth. The baby will grow at the expense of the mother if food is deficient. Low levels of vitamin A, iron, zinc, selenium and vitamin D in the mother's diet (Venter 2006) and atopic reactions by the pregnant woman (Jones *et al.* 2002) may later show in a reduction of immune function and allergic sensitisation in the young baby. However, Cox (2006) showed there was no evidence for special diets in pregnancy. At birth, the baby can depend on colostrum: a thin, yellowish fluid which is particularly valuable for the establishment of lactobacilli in the gut, and contains less fat and energy but more secretory IgA immunoglobulin than later breast milk. Mature breast milk, produced at ten to fourteen days after birth, is unique in that its composition varies over the course of a feed, a day and the period of lactation. Lactose is the principal carbohydrate of mature breast milk, providing about 39 per cent of the energy for the baby. Proteins composing 60 per cent whey to 40 per cent casein are particularly easily digested, and predominantly long-chain fatty acids provide 50 per cent of all energy requirements until the age of six months, when the gut physiology is matured and weaning to solids can commence. Breast milk also contains a number of anti-infective properties such as macrophages, IgA, lysozyme, lactoferrin, interferon and bifidus factor, which appear to protect the infant from respiratory and gastrointestinal infections in the first few months of life (Rudolf and Leucene 1999). Furber and Thomson (2006) explored breastfeeding attitudes and found that social, psychological, cultural and economic factors influenced mothers: older women, those in the higher socio-economic groups and with good family support were the most successful. They suggest that mothers are influenced by their friends, knowledge of breastfeeding and the way they themselves were fed as babies. Bottle-feeding of infant formula is a safe alternative, if all the hygiene and preparation instructions are followed; however, cow's full fat pasteurised milk is not suitable for infants under one year, as the sodium content is too high and the iron content is too low for their nutritional requirements (Wilkinson and Walker 2007). Current UK recommendation is for formula milk rather than full fat cow's milk to be consumed from six months until the first birthday. The composition of all infant milk formulas in the UK complies with government guidelines.

Weaning presents an early challenge to both mother and child. Different tastes and textures have to be experienced gradually in order that the child will accept a varied diet and thus the range of nutrients for optimal growth. Formula milk alone, although continuing as an important source of nourishment for the growing baby, will not provide enough energy for the four- to six-month-old child; by this age their stores of iron and zinc, important for red blood cell function and immune system response, will be low. Lumps in food are needed to stimulate chewing and development of the jaw, which is vital for the later function of speech (www.eatwell.gov.uk/ages). Food refusal, faddy feeding and mealtime battles are common at the one- to three-year stage, but if sweet drinks and crisps are not offered as substitutes for meals, children will eventually accept a range of nutritious foods to keep them healthy as they grow through their early childhood. Even some of the more restricted menus, such as baked beans, bread, bananas and fish fingers, are better than canned fizzy drinks and salty snacks. All children, particularly those under the age of two years, need some fat in the diet to give energy and vitamin A, D and E supplies: a low fat diet and skimmed milk are not suitable at this young age. From the age of two to five years, fruit and vegetables – the five portion advice – should be encouraged to increase fibre in the diet and ensure regular bowel function (Wilkinson and Walker 2007).

The nutritional standards requirements for schools was abandoned in 1980 (Holden and MacDonald 2000), but in 1999 the Department for Education and Employment spearheaded the primary schools national strategy for healthy eating (DFEE 1999 and Robinson 2006). This, plus the intense media promotion of healthy foods, is having an effect of raising awareness of the importance of a balanced diet. However, there is still a widespread cafeteria-style school lunch of a snack-type nature, even at five years of age when children enter the education system. Children can still be seen to purchase 'tasty' food snacks that are high in fat and sugar, processed and packaged, and many schoolchildren do not eat breakfast and 'graze' in the evening. Free school meals in 2007 are only available for children whose low income parents draw family credit. However, health promotion initiatives have increased in schools, healthy eating is included in the National Curriculum and promoted by high profile chefs such as Jamie Oliver, and school nurses are involved in the school day with children to encourage sensible eating and exercise opportunities (Peate and Whiting 2006). Those eating excessive amounts of these high-calorie/low-nutrient diets can become obese, with subsequent long-term development of low self-esteem and muscular, skeletal and cardiovascular pathologies. Obesity is evident in 30 per cent of school-aged children (see www.healthline.com) and the development of mature onset diabetes in the young (MODY) is increasing (Haines *et al.* 2007). Those pre-pubescent children eating small amounts of low-calorie foods, often with few nutrients, in order to stay slim, or who come from families on a low income where food choice is limited, may also find that emotional and intellectual development deteriorates (Holden and MacDonald 2000). Magnusson (2005) suggests that balanced management is best between a diet which is manipulated for either calorie control, fat reduction, reduction of specific foods such as crisps or increase of specific foods such as fruit and vegetables, and an exercise regime where there is a structured programme of increasing lifestyle activity and reducing sedentary behaviour.

Adolescence is a time of rapid development. To sustain this rate of growth the metabolism speeds up, ensuring that nutrients are processed quickly and energy released. As a result appetite increases, especially for foods with high sugar content. It is not unusual for this age group (boys in particular) to feel the need for snacks, even before and after their main meals. 'Grazing' food can be a physiologically healthy behaviour; the stomach is given small amounts to digest at any one time in response to a desire to eat. Intake responds to a reduced blood sugar that stimulates the 'hunger centre' in the brain. Holden and MacDonald (2000) identify vegetarianism, teenage pregnancy, sports and athletic training, smoking, drinking alcohol and slimming diets to have profound effect on long-term health for this age group. The adolescent, however, lives in the 'immediate' world and healthy eating behaviour may not fit with his or her daily routine and peer group norms.

The need for temperature control

Humans are homeothermic. They regulate their body temperature, created by their metabolic rate, in relation to their external environment. This regulation is controlled by peripheral thermo-receptors in the skin and central thermo-receptors in the anterior hypothalamus, which monitor the temperature of the blood. As the blood passes through the hypothalamus, information is relayed to the autonomic nervous and endocrine systems for responses that return body temperature to the 'normal set point' so that enzyme activity in all the body cells can proceed.

The 'normal set point' in childhood reflects a decreasing basic metabolic rate (BMR) as the child grows. The body temperature of the three-month-old child is 37.5 °C, whereas at thirteen years it is 36.6 °C (Wong *et al.* 2003). Even as the temperature regulatory mechanisms mature through childhood, babies and small children are highly susceptible to temperature fluctuations, as they produce more heat per kilogram of body weight than older children. Changes in environmental temperature, increased activity, crying, emotional upset and infections all cause a higher and more rapid increase in the younger child. The younger the child the less able he or she is to vocalise the feeling of hot or cold or to do something about it.

All children may also become too cold. Small individuals who do not have warm clothes and warm homes will not grow if the temperature of their environment is consistently low. They will use much of the energy from their food intake to generate heat (metabolic rate) and leave no spare calories for tissue growth. The smaller the child, the larger the surface area for heat loss in relation to body mass. The head of a small child is relatively larger in proportion to the rest of the body, and covering the head in a cold environment conserves heat for growth. Schoolchildren may experience a sequence of small growth spurts and at times be relatively thin with minimal body fat. At the swimming pool, for example, where children enjoy jumping in and out of the water as they play, thin children may become cold more quickly than their fatter friends who have an insulation layer beneath their skin.

The need for activity, rest and sleep

As children grow they develop more gross motor abilities and coordination, which allow them to further explore their world and take part in simple physical games. Exercise is essential for muscle development and tone, refinement of balance, gaining strength and endurance, and stimulating body functions and metabolic processes (Wong 2003).

Most infants enjoy being free of their clothes and allowed to kick and wriggle on a blanket on the floor, or to splash and kick in the bath. Turner (2002) describes the sequential stages of motor development where the baby moves from prone to sitting to standing positions, and the need for the child to acquire these new skills by trial and error, practise and application. Children should be encouraged to develop flexibility with their bodies through having the opportunity to move freely and safely.

During the school years, children take part in physical exercises in order to acquire timing and concentration in the more complex physical activities. They need space to run, jump, skip and climb in safety to do this, and they need the positive reinforcement of experiencing an increasingly efficient use of their body. Fitness in children can be measured by their cardiovascular endurance, blood pressure, blood lipid profile, fatness and glucose tolerance – their metabolic fitness (Boreham and Riddoch 2001). Improved fitness can be attained by engaging in aerobic activities for twenty to twenty-five minutes three times per week where the heart rate is maintained at 75 per cent of maximum. Children can be encouraged to be active through physical movements they enjoy, such as football and dancing. Activities that stress the skeleton against gravity will encourage uptake of calcium from the diet and thus strengthen the weight-bearing bones. School-age children enjoy competition in sport; however, their carers must be mindful of teaching proper skills appropriately, and matching activities to their physical abilities in order that excess sporting activity does not injure developing muscles and bones.

Older children who do not engage in physical pursuits, and are praised for being quiet when they play with computers and video games for long periods of time each day, are missing a critical period for the establishment of healthy body systems for later adult life.

All children need to sleep; it is then that they grow and the repair of body tissues occurs. The total number of hours in a twenty-four hour period should range from eight to ten, but need not necessarily be taken in one session; for example, children in hot climates sleep in the afternoons and stay up late with their parents in the cooler evenings. Many circumstances affect a child's ability to sleep well: they may not have regular routines before bed, they may be anxious about being safe, they may be hungry or they may be too hot or cold. When children fall into 'deep sleep' it is then that their growth hormone is activated from the pituitary gland and released in pulses into the blood stream: they need a sleep 'cycle' of an hour for this to be effective. Growth hormone stimulates the growth plate in the long bones of the skeleton to make new bone.

Physiology knowledge in practice

Scenario 1

You are observing a school nurse advising a group of teenagers on physical harm from smoking, drinking excess alcohol and having sexual relationships with multiple partners. What basic information would you expect him/her to give?

Some pointers:

Smoking

- Nicotine affects brain function as it stimulates vasoconstriction by directly activating ganglionic sympathetic neurons and also prompts release of large amounts of adrenaline and nor-adrenaline from the adrenal medulla. This raises blood pressure and pulse. It has a cocaine-like effect on the brain function to produce a feeling of elation and increased physical activity ability. It is a fat soluble molecule that passes through the brain/blood barrier.
- The smoke decreases the function of the cilia lining the respiratory tract and increases the number of irritant particles in the airways.
- The tar stays in the lungs and occludes gas exchange in the airways.

Alcohol

- Alcohol affects brain function as it is a fat soluble substance that can cross the brain/blood barrier and give a relaxed feeling. In excess it is a central nervous system depressant as it affects the reticular formation leading to motor and intellectual dysfunction.
- At moderate levels of 20 mg/100 ml, it has been shown to have a beneficial effect on the cardiovascular system as it raises the plasma high density lipoprotein/cholesterol levels. Females are recommended no more than 2 units (16 gm) per day and males 3 units (24 gm). A unit is a glass of wine or half a pint of beer. New directions are that all pregnant females should abstain for nine months, however, there is the alternative view that a small amount daily does no harm. Prenatal exposure leads to foetal alcohol syndrome which includes growth retardation, cognitive impairment, facial anomalies and ocular disturbances and failure of some brain regions to develop (McCance and Heuther 2006).
- It is absorbed from the digestive tract in the stomach and in excess irritates the stomach lining resulting in a chronic gastritis. Alcohol is a poison: as it passes through the liver it is metabolised to acetaldehyde. We all have different genetic ability to detoxify alcohol in the liver. In excess it will damage the hepatocytes. These filtering cells can regenerate but the surrounding liver connective tissue – the scar – regenerates faster and the result is that the liver becomes fatty and the scar tissue shrinks and obstructs the flow through of blood. This causes a rise in hepatic portal blood pressure.
- Alcohol's effect on nutrition is that it reduces the concentration of magnesium in the body and also vitamin B6, thiamine and phosphorous.

Sexual activity

- Sexually transmitted diseases give rise to pelvic inflammatory disease, infertility, ectopic pregnancy, chronic pelvic pain, neonatal morbidity and mortality. They are prevalent in all social classes.
- Adolescent risk taking behaviour, such as poor use of condoms, increases the risk of infection due to the immature cervix in the female and lack of full immunity status.
- Need to give contraceptive advice.

Scenario 2

You are observing a health visitor at a new client home appointment with a single mother and her two-year-old child. What safety information would you expect to hear?

Some pointers:

- Consider the kitchen, living room/space, bedroom and garden/ outside area. Think of all the dangers for a small child and how they can be minimised. Some areas might contain wires and plugs, open space access, stairs/steps, fires and hot appliances and medications. Find a picture of a typical room and design your own teaching aid for a mother who has low educational ability or has poor English use. You can label the picture and have the clues on the back.
- Do the same with a road scene/play area/park. Consider such items as the 'green cross code', safe places to play in the park, helmet for the tricycle, reins to control the child near the road, safe use of the push chair and the danger of water.

Extend your knowledge

Reilly *et al.* (2005) discuss the phenomenon of obesity in their article entitled 'Early life risk factors for obesity in children'. They suggest that professionals need to monitor fatness and consider factors such as the early life risk factors, the economic situation of the family, their educational level, their social situation and the psychological effects of becoming/being fat.

Consider a family of children aged nine months, two years, five years, ten years and sixteen years – all girls. What are normal ranges of measurement for them? What economic factors might be important to consider and why? What educational factors could be impacting? Think about the different social groups and how these children may have become too fat and how it might affect their overall development in the next year if intervention is not successful.

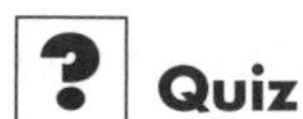

Quiz

1. What are the five ECM principles?
2. What are the six UNICEF categories for children's health?
3. What are the three fundamental concepts for considering child development?
4. How can genetics explain the relative differences of children in a Year Three class?
5. Give three environmental effects that might explain a three-year-old child failing to thrive.
6. Why are children more vulnerable to accidents than adults?
7. What type of accident would you expect in the adolescent age group and why?
8. How might you recognise an abused baby, child or adolescent?
9. Why do all children need a secure attachment?
10. Describe the stages of healthy social cognitive development.
11. What is the childhood immunisation schedule for the UK?
12. Why may parents not wish to have their children vaccinated?
13. Why is breast milk best for human babies and how long is it recommended a mother breastfeeds her baby?
14. What are main food group recommendations in a healthy diet?
15. What may prevent an adolescent eating healthily?
16. Why might a child become obese?
17. Why is there a risk of hypothermia in babies?
18. What physical activities would you suggest for a family outing with children of six, eight and ten years?
19. How might children's fitness be measured?
20. Why do children need to have adequate sleep?

Further reading

Department for Education and Employment (2006) *Framework for the Assessment of Children in Need and their Families*, London: The Stationery Office.

Department of Health (2003) *Every Child Matters: Change for Children*, available online at www.everychildmatters.gov.uk, accessed July 2007.

Department of Health (2004) *National Service Framework (NSF) for Children, Young People and Maternity Services (England)*. Available online at www.everychildmatters.gov.uk/publications, accessed July 2007.

Milupa, website available at www.milupaaptamil4hcps.co.uk/immunesystem, accessed July 2007.

Chapter 2

The skeletal system

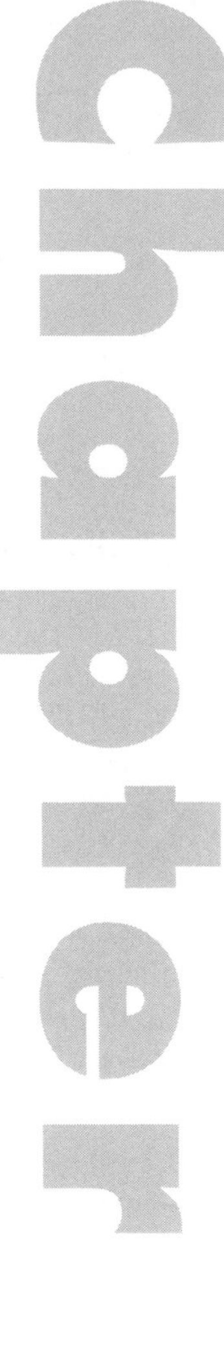

- Embryology
- The changing skeleton
- Growth in height
- Genetic inheritance
- Hormones of growth
- Exercise
- Nature–nurture
- Strength
- Physical activity play
- Body shape changes

THE DEVELOPING SKELETON changes and moulds as forces exert pressure on it during the individual's muscle activity, movement of other parts of the skeleton and the individual's genetic programme. This occurs, not only in childhood, but throughout the age span. The skeletal system is the best documented of all the systems in children; its internal and external changes – 'bone age' – are recognised anatomically.

Embryology

The skeleton commences its development early in foetal life; the maternal calcium stores will become depleted if this mineral is not ingested to support the foetal changes. At the end of the fourth week of gestation, embryonic connective tissue in the region of the future skeleton shows signs of differentiation. Primitive cells become more closely packed and lay down a cartilage matrix rich in chondroitin sulphate. At six weeks of foetal life the embryonic vertebrae are forming from the mesoderm, and by the eighth week primary ossification is evident at antenatal scan (see Figure 2.1). The cells round the developing cartilage form two layers; those of the outer layer change to fibroblasts, and the inner ones to cartilage and the perichondrium. Layers of cells are then added superficially as the bones grow.

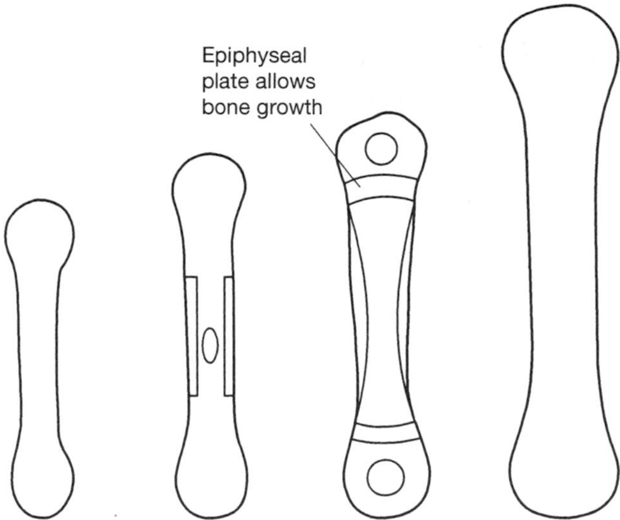
Epiphyseal
plate allows
bone growth

Figure 2.1 Primary and secondary ossification centres

Two groups of bone cells work antagonistically through life to maintain the skeleton. Osteoblasts are modified fibroblasts which have collagen fibres deposited round them, calcium salts then accumulate here to increase bone size. Osteoclasts, developed from the bone marrow stem cells, then continually shape bone by removing excess material.

Ossification of many bones occurs in the second month of foetal life. The clavicle and bones of the skull vault ossify 'in membrane' as blood vessels penetrate the area and bring in osteoblasts and osteoclasts. Other bones ossify as the connective tissue converts to a cartilage template and then to bone. These starting points for bone ossification are called primary centres, and appear in different bones at different times (Jenkins *et al.* 2007, Neill and Knowles 2004).

The changing skeleton

Skeletal age is best measured at the left wrist and hand. An individual is compared to standard radiography (TW2 method). This is a score of the stage of development of the twenty bones of the wrist and hand. The score is relatively subjective and depends on the presence of bones and epiphyses, and the relationship of their size, shape and markings. Girls are two years ahead of boys, but carpal bones are not visible under two years for either sex. The vertebral spine has two primary curves present at birth, but normally by adolescence four vertebral curves are evident; the cervical (lordotic), the thoracic (primary curve), the lumbar (lordotic) and the sacral (primary curve) (see Figure 2.2).

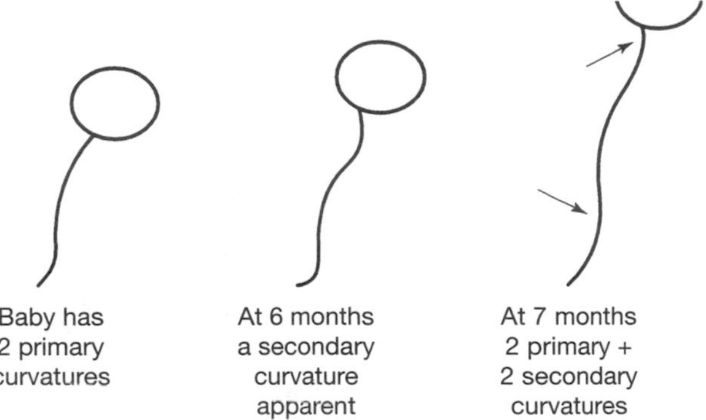
Baby has
2 primary
curvatures
At 6 months
a secondary
curvature
apparent
At 7 months
2 primary +
2 secondary
curvatures

Figure 2.2 Development of the four vertebral curves

The infant's head shows the skull bones to be thin and the facial bones small. The jaw is small at birth with usually no teeth, but grows until puberty when adult proportions are apparent (Figure 2.3). Resuscitation in children under seven years of age demands a different technique to that of adults, as the head and neck anatomy results in relatively high positions of larynx and trachea and the rib cage is more compliant. Small children have small facial sinuses which do not reach adult size until the age of ten/twelve years. Listen to a group at play in your local infant school and you will not be able to distinguish the individual voices of these small people who uniformly have high-pitched voices that only their mothers recognise. It will only be when they finish their growth at puberty that the genetics of their family will have been expressed. By then their faces will have developed the full number of sinuses and likeness of their parents, and their voices will show individual characteristics.

As the sinuses increase in size, so infections are less able to become lodged in small crevices. Together with the developed ability to coordinate in order to blow one's nose and improving immune response, constant runny noses should become a thing of the past and ear and throat infections reduced.

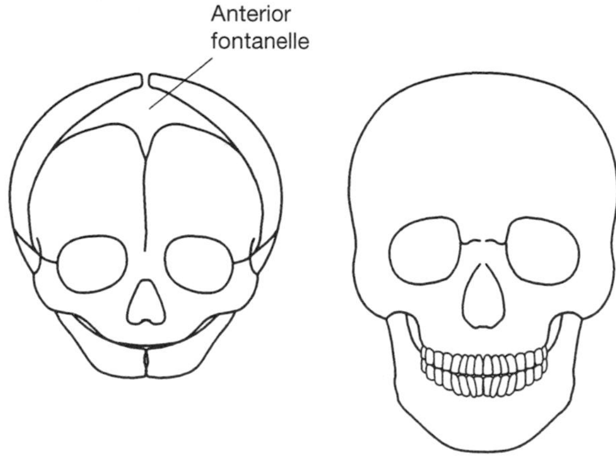

Figure 2.3 Bone structure in the infant and adolescent skull

Growth in height

Growth is influenced by normal inheritance, physiological age, normal variation in nutritional status, health, hormonal status and antenatal history.

Voss *et al.* (1998), in the Wessex Growth Study, found that although birth weight and parental height were the major biological predictors of growth at school entry, social and environmental factors have a powerful effect. They found psychological deprivation, large families and a father who was unemployed to be the most frequent variables. Predicted height can be approximately calculated in children after the age of two years. The Child Growth Foundation charts for children from birth to eighteen (www.fph.org.uk) have calculations on each chart for identifying the adult height potential. Until then there is some readjusting of size to genetically determined growth rates; some large babies will adjust down and some small babies will adjust up.

Genetic inheritance

The sequencing and timing of growth is influenced by the genes, and these affect different groups differently. At birth, the reason for relatively advanced skeletal development in females is the retarding action of the genes on the Y chromosome in the male. Afro-Caribbean children grow faster in the first two years of life and their bone density is higher at all ages; males and females of all races show different tissue growth at puberty.

Growth shows individual variation; growth spurts occur in a biphasic pattern for both height and weight. It is distinctive in primates; males and females show different patterns, and different parts of the body have different growth curves. For example, the lymph system is the fastest growing tissue and the reproductive system the slowest in childhood (Tanner 1989). Growth shows a series of changes. Specialisation of various parts of the body and alteration of body form includes the incidental destruction and death of cells and tissues and substitution. For example, bone develops from cartilage and modification of the shape of the skeleton occurs under the influence of the sex hormones testosterone and oestrogen. While growth rate is different for the various body tissues, one part may be controlled by the other, for example growth hormone secretion and bone length. Growth is continuous; the building and destruction in the moulding process of the skeleton occurs throughout life.

Body proportions change over the period of childhood. There is an increase in the relative length of the legs in relation to height as the child moves into puberty resulting in a decreasing ratio of sitting height to stature. The body mass reduces in relation to surface area: 50 per cent from the age of five years to adult status. This is reflected in the overall reduction of basic metabolic rate (BMR) over the childhood years. However, parents will report periods of rapid growth and periods of little change in height – the 'Christmas tree pattern'. Peak height velocity, the maximum growth rate, is seen in the adolescent spurt.

Growth factors are usually proteins and may be produced locally in tissues – pancrine factors – or further away within the endocrine system. Growth factors act on specific protein receptors in the lipid layers of the plasma membranes of the cells to stimulate a chemical signal to the nucleus – the autocrine effect. When the cell is stimulated, amino acids are taken up into the cytoplasm to form protein, and thus growth occurs.

In childhood, growth hormone (GH) levels rise eight to nine times in twenty-four hours for ten to twenty minutes. Usually the bursts are at night when the child descends into deep-phase sleep. GH is increased in adolescence, stimulated by the increase in sex hormone production. GH needs an 'intermediate' chemical in order for it to be activated. Somatomedian is secreted by the proliferative cells in the growth plate (Figure 2.4) as well as the liver, which is the main source of this hormone.

Hormones of growth

Many hormones (chemical messengers) are involved in growth – some of them more involved in the developing foetus such as prolactin, chorion gonadotrophic hormone and placenta lactogen, whereas others have ongoing effect.

The hypothalamus, the centre of endocrine control in the brain, is thought to keep the growth curve to the genetically determined pathway, and it is interesting that a child who suffers periods of poor feeding will usually 'catch up'. The hypothalamus interacts with the pituitary which lies beneath it to influence the coordination of the

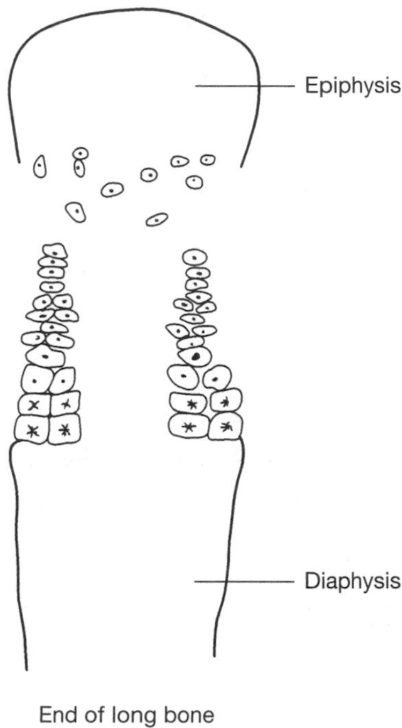

Figure 2.4 The growth plate

whole endocrine system. Peripheral nerves also appear to play a part in exerting a nutritive or 'trophic' effect by secreting some chemical to the tissue they supply. If a hand nerve is cut, the nail does not grow well until the nerve regenerates; sensory nerves appear to influence this phenomenon more than motor nerves. Local growth is controlled by chalones which are chemicals that balance the cell division and differentiation phases in tissue growth; they are formed by actively dividing cells. They are also secreted by cells adjacent to dividing cells in their cell membranes to control cell spacing. Age of tissue, and its mitotic ability, influence chalone secretion, thus the growing child replaces damaged tissue quickly after injury.

Growth hormone, somatotropin, is a protein which is secreted from the anterior pituitary gland. It causes most body cells to increase in size and divide. Its major targets are the bones, cartilage, skeletal muscles and epiphyseal plates. It does not affect the brain, adrenals and gonads; the sexual changes of adolescence rely on increased sex hormone secretion for development of secondary sexual characteristics. Growth hormone is an anabolic hormone. This means it promotes protein synthesis and the use of fats for cellular fuel in order to conserve glucose. It competes for the same cell membrane receptors as insulin and is opposed by cortisol. Its secretion is stimulated by a lowering of blood sugar levels, food intake, exercise and injury (especially burns). It is also controlled directly by a second messenger system, the somatomedians, which are insulin-like growth factors, produced by the liver, kidneys and muscles. Children who have liver or kidney malfunction have poor growth.

GH affects how nutrients are metabolised:

- stimulates the uptake of amino acids from the blood and their incorporation into proteins and the reduction of protein breakdown for cellular energy release;
- stimulates the uptake of the mineral sulphur needed for the synthesis of chondroitin sulphate into the cartilage matrix;
- stimulates the mobilisation of fats from adipose tissue for transport to cells, thus increasing the blood levels of fatty acids for cell uptake and energy release;
- reduces glucose uptake by cells for energy release, thus increasing blood glucose levels.

It is regulated by two hypothalamic hormones with antagonistic effects. GHRH (growth hormone-releasing hormone) stimulates its release, activated by feedback blood levels of GH and somatomedian. GHIH (growth hormone-inhibiting hormone) opposes GHRH; it is a very powerful hormone which blocks other pituitary effects in the body such as gastrointestinal and pancreatic function. These hormones have a diurnal cycle, with the steeper rise during deep wave sleep.

Another endocrine gland, the thyroid, produces thyroxin which accelerates the rate of cellular metabolism throughout the body. It is the regulator of growth and development; it stimulates skeletal growth and the maturation of the nervous system but inhibits that of the reproductive system. It does this by stimulating enzymes concerned with glucose oxidation, and increases metabolic rate and oxygen consumption thus increasing body heat. Thyroxin (T3 and T4) binds to the plasma proteins produced by the liver which transport it to target tissue receptors. Plasma enzymes convert T4 to T3, and then remove all the thyroxin to the mitochondria and nucleus of the cell.

The thyroid also produces calcitonin, a hormone which antagonises parathyroid. It acts on the skeleton by inhibiting bone reabsorption and the release of ionic calcium from the bony matrix. It stimulates calcium uptake from the blood and its incorporation into the bone matrix by the osteoblasts. It increases the excretion of calcium and phosphate ions by the kidney. Raised blood calcium (over 20 per cent) stimulates its release.

Another set of glands, the parathyroids which lie behind the thyroid gland in the neck area, are triggered by a decrease in blood calcium levels, and are inhibited by raised levels. Parathyroid hormone increases ionic calcium levels by stimulating release from the skeleton, which results in the activation of the bone reabsorbing cells, the osteoclasts, to release calcium and phosphates to the blood. It acts on the kidney tubules to reabsorb calcium ions and magnesium and decrease the retention of phosphate. It increases absorption of calcium, phosphates and magnesium by intestinal mucosa cells. This action is enhanced by the parathyroid effect on vitamin D activation to 1,25-dihydroxycholecal-ciferol in the kidney.

Yet another pair of glands, the adrenals, are activated by the hypothalamus cortisol activating hormone, which stimulates the pituitary to secrete ACTH (adrenocorticotropic hormone). The adrenal gland produces three hormones from its cortex:

- Glucocorticoids – 95 per cent of which are cortisol – influence metabolism of most body cells. Bursts occur in a pattern over the day, peaking in the morning and reducing towards the evening. It is regulated by eating and physical activity and affected by stress. As the sympathetic nervous system overrides the inhibitory action of an elevated cortisol level on CRH release, ACTH continues to be released and further raises the cortisol levels. Stressed children do not grow, as they have a chronic raised metabolic rate. Cortisol also converts non-carbohydrates, that is fats and proteins, to glucose for energy, thus reducing the availability of these nutrients for tissue development. High levels of glucocorticoids depress cartilage and bone formation and reduce muscle mass. Chronically stressed children will use all their nutrients for energy release rather than for tissue building.
- Mineralcorticoids are responsible for the electrolyte composition of body fluids. Aldosterone is the major mineralcorticoid which regulates sodium and potassium. It increases absorption of sodium and thus has effect on the blood pressure and blood volume. It is controlled by the rennin-angiotensin-aldosterone pathway which is activated by stimuli such as dehydration, low

blood sodium, haemorrhage and low filtration pressures in the kidney.

- Androgens are activated by ACTH. They stimulate metabolic processes, especially those concerned with protein synthesis and muscle growth. In females they contribute to the development of libido and are converted to oestrogen by body tissues. They sustain the growth of axilla and pubic hair at puberty and contribute to the development of 'teenage spots' in males and females.

The pancreas, a gland with endocrine and exocrine function, produces insulin hormone pulses at 13-minute intervals; this allows a constant flow of glucose to transfer into most cells of the body. The cells then make ATP (adenosine triphosphate – an energy source) which they use to pull amino-acids from the blood to build proteins and thus support growth. Any stimulus that raises blood sugar will have this effect on the pancreas, such as the ingestion of food, production of adrenaline, growth hormone, thyroxin or cortisols. The production of insulin is halted by somatostatin which is secreted by both the hypothalamus, the pancreas D cells and throughout the gastrointestinal tract. The major affect of somatostatin is to inhibit insulin and glucagon local to the pancreas where most of it is secreted. It also inhibits digestive function by reducing gut motility, gastric secretion and pancreatic endocrine function and absorption at the gut mucosa, therefore pacing foodstuff conversion.

Finally the gonads, producing testosterone (in the male) and oestrogen (in the female), show rising levels at puberty. In males this hormone effect leads to the increase in bone growth and density and skeletal muscle size and mass. Testosterone boosts the basic metabolic rate at all stages of the male child's life. At puberty, energy needs are enormous – teenage boys will snack before and after normal family meals!

Oestrogen, in the female, also has an anabolic effect in puberty, particularly on the female secondary sexual charateristics. The breasts grow, subcutaneous fat increases, the pelvis widens and calcium is facilitated into the skeleton. Oestrogen also supports her skeletal growth spurt until levels are high enough to close the epiphyseal plates and stop long bone growth and thus height. Low oestrogen levels have been found to have a powerful effect in offsetting the positive bone mass accumulation promoted by calcium in the diet and by weight bearing exercise.

Diet calcium for bone growth

The recommended calcium intake over childhood rises with age. The reference nutrient intake (RNI) is set in the UK at 700 mg for the adult population. The proportion of calcium uptake compared to body weight is highest in the term foetus, where 300 mg calcium passes through the placenta each day. The teenager requires 800–1,000 mgs. Children from seven to ten years are recommended to need 550 mg (Geissler and Powers 2005). Calcium and vitamin D are linked; calcium levels in the blood require vitamin D for intestinal absorption, maintenance of circulating calcium levels and bone mineralisation. Adequate levels of sunshine on children's skin in the summer months will ensure they do not need dietary supplementation of vitamin D.

Exercise

Genetic factors account for 60 per cent of performance, but physical activity that stresses bones, nutritional sufficiency especially of calcium and vitamin D, hormone effect and drug use may all have a bearing on the achievement of peak bone mass. Physical activity of three hours per week, which starts before the pre-pubertal growth spurt, in activities such as gymnastics and football/handball increases the lean mass of skeletal muscle. This tissue will give maximum tension on developing bones to ensure optimal mineral mass accrual. As boys spend a longer time in the pre-pubertal period they grow longer extremities and increase their bone mass to 20 per cent more than girls by the age of sixteen to seventeen years. Weight bearing sport activities for both sexes before puberty generate compressive forces on the epiphiseal growth plates of the long bones which lead to bigger bones, better ossified lumbar spine and a femoral bone mass that lasts for life. The establishment of a maximum bone density in the years of growth is vital to long-term skeletal health; 90 per cent of bone mass has been laid down by the end of puberty; 25 per cent of the adult bone mass is attained in the two-year period of the growth spurt (eleven to thirteen years for girls and twelve to fourteen years for boys) (Rodriguez 2006, Watts *et al.* 2005). Peak bone mass is difficult to determine, however, because different bones achieve their peak bone density at different times. However, all factors interrelate: for example, maximum physical activity with absence of normal oestrogen levels in adolescent females results in a weakened skeleton, although mechanical loading remains the pre-eminent factor for skeletal integrity (Bailey and Martin 1994).

Changes in bone due to exercise

The key variable between skeletal loading and bone mass is the mechanical strain placed on the bone. Rodriguez (2006) found that intensity of load is more important than duration in children. Tensile, compressive, shear, bending and torsion stress have osteogenic potential. Changes in the internal bone strain appear to activate osteoblasts, which will change the dynamic balance from bone loss to bone formation. In regular strain – repeated vigorous physical activity – there is a gain in bone formation. This increase in bone mass then reduces the load over the larger bone, and eventually balance is regained between bone loss and bone gain at the higher bone mass. However, not all activity will promote bone growth; the activity needs to be weight bearing, thus football produces good bone growth in many skeletal bones, whereas swimming and horse riding do not.

Early skeletal maturation can show an observable advantage in children being stronger and faster and with higher oxygen uptake than their 'younger' peers. Many of these children are also advanced in sexual development, as the hormones that stimulate growth in bone muscle also affect the sexual organs. This effect is most pronounced during puberty rather than before. Before puberty GH is responsible for bone and somatic growth, whereas during puberty the sex hormone, testosterone, effect becomes superimposed on it.

Nature–nurture

Genetic correlation has been found in bone mineral content, grip, strength, activity, height and triceps skin-fold thickness in three generations (Kahn *et al.* 1994). However, more recently there appears to be considerable evidence to support physical activity as the important non-inherited factor. Branca (1999) found that physical activity such as walking, rather than cycling or swimming, increased all the children's bone mass in her sample. Siranda and Pate (2001) studied physical activity in schools and found that 5 to 20 per cent of daily activity requirements were achieved in moderate intensity playground games between classroom sessions, but this was dependent on the different cultures, age groups and sex of the young people they studied.

Strength

The amount of habitual physical activity effect has on height is nil. Exercise has most effect on body weight where there is a decrease in body fat and increase in muscle mass and bone mineralisation, but not in bone maturation. Morris *et al.* (1997), in their study of nine to ten-year-olds, found that the children gained lean body mass and increased their shoulder, knee and grip strength, and also increased their bone mineral density after three thirty-minute strengthening sessions per week. Body composition has a significant influence on the physiological response to exercise as the muscle mass (motor) has to move the body fat (baggage). Small children spend most of their time in short bursts of activity which are largely anaerobic.

This activity ability increases with age, but changes are more than can be ascribed to growth and will be exercise related. Strength develops in direct relationship to neural influence, with males showing an advanced gender difference from the age of three years and increasing most during puberty under the influence of testosterone. As muscle size increases so does strength. The number of muscle fibres is fixed at birth, but as they hypertrophy they grow in size; males have 42 per cent muscle at five years and 53 per cent at seventeen years. Interestingly, there is no change in this same proportion of muscle in females as they move through puberty. Muscle structure is determined at birth by the genetic inheritance. As muscles mature their ability to contract is more efficient. Together with their growth in size, so strength increases. Patel *et al.* (2006) studied high intensity exercise in children and found that they recovered more quickly than adults. They explained that children's muscles are different as they have less muscle mass with less type 2 fibres so generate lower absolute power in exercise and have less muscle fibre fatigue. They have better oxidative than glycolytic pathways of sugar metabolism so they generate less muscle activity by-products, such as lactic acid, and remove them faster. Resistance training for children is useful as it helps females to put down calcium in bones and thus lessen the impact of osteoporosis in later life; it also reduces the possibility of physical injury and produces a healthier blood fat/protein profile.

Activity stimulates the secretion of GH to mobilise fats for energy and develop lean muscle mass. In females who are very active, sex hormones are reduced as body fat reduces and muscle mass increases; thus puberty can be delayed.

Children produce a greater amount of heat relative to body mass when they exercise, and they sweat less. They rely on a greater cutaneous blood flow to lose heat from their greater surface area; toddlers have subcutaneous fat to insulate them. A small child's head surface is 20 per cent of his or her total body surface and is an important consideration in managing temperature control. The young child adjusts more slowly to hot environments and alternatively becomes hypothermic more quickly, as they lose heat from their larger skin surface area.

Physical activity play

Pellegrini and Smith (1998) propose that physical play, although it is enjoyable, has an immediate developmental function for physical, cognitive and social skills. They suggest three distinct phases of physical activity.

The first is a stage of 'rhythmic stereotype' which peaks in infancy. Children at this stage strive to improve control of specific and gross motor movement patterns. This activity peaks at six months, and children can spend up to 40 per cent of their time kicking their legs, smacking their play arch or other similar movements. The onset of this is controlled by neuromuscular maturation. This type of play modifies or eliminates irrelevant synapse formation. As the neurone pathways mature, infants begin to use pathways that they have developed in a more goal-directed way to manipulate toys or feeding bottles/cups, for example.

The second stage, exercise play, can be seen in the pre-school child. Here children develop their strength and endurance. They can now commence more intensive motor training as locomotion occurs. Gross motor development declines at the age of five years and only accounts for 20 per cent of their physical activity. Pre-school children run, flee, wrestle, chase, jump, push and pull, lift and climb. Muscle strength, central nervous function and metabolic capacity improve skills ability and economy of movement. Exercise will have the effect of increasing muscle fibre differentiation and cerebellar synaptogenesis. The eventual outcome will be to demonstrate fine motor control. The more exercise that is taken, the more endurance and strength are developed. Climbing frames, walking, riding bikes and kicking balls are all activities of play that will develop the neuromuscular pathway and remodel the skeleton. Children of this age need hourly bouts of activity each day. They also need to develop confidence in movement through reasonable physical challenges and take risks. Over-protection severely limits the child's opportunities to engage in exciting opportunities – such as splashing in puddles for the toddler age group. May *et al.* (2006) explain how this preparation to respond to reasonable challenges helps them eventually to become physically competent and safe.

The third stage, rough and tumble play, is seen most clearly in mid-childhood. This play also has a social animal dimension in the development of dominance function and fighting skills. Wood and Attfield (2006) warn how this can go beyond socially acceptable behaviour – the 'super hero' play which needs adult management and the rough and tumble play that goes beyond a safe or appropriate activity. Children try to come to terms with and master the plural cultures of home, school and society by being 'powerful' in their adult dominated world. From the age of six to ten years exercise play declines to 13 per cent of the child's activity. At nine to ten years, running, walking fast, games, sports and cycling are enjoyed. Males indulge in wrestling, grappling, kicking and tumbling; this is aggressive but playful, although they will often get hurt. This activity can be seen in 4 per cent of four-year-olds, 7 to 8 per cent of six- to ten-year-olds, 10 per cent of seven- to eleven-year-olds, 4 per cent of eleven- to thirteen-year-olds and 2 per cent of boys at fourteen. Children of this age are testing their strength against their peers and trying out social dominance by physical means.

Body shape changes

Parts of the body grow at different rates and have growth spurts at different times; thus the child changes radically from stage to stage of childhood (Figure 2.5). At birth the infant head is of the proportion 1:4; in the adult it is 1:8. The infant lower limbs are 15 per cent of the total body weight compared to 30 per cent in the adult. As growth proceeds, the centre of gravity moves down from the twelfth thoracic vertebra to the fifth lumbar by adult height. Thus the child's wide stance is responding to carrying a head that is twice the size of the adult, on legs that are half the length, and not necessarily responding to nappy padding. Black children, however, have relatively longer limbs, faster developing muscles, and may hold their head up, sit up and walk earlier than white children. The infant head circumference is the same as the chest; that of the abdomen is greater than both until the age of two years when the pelvic bones grow and allow abdominal contents to drop down into it. Also at this age, the neck becomes more obvious as the thorax and shoulder girdle also descend. Up to this time the ribs lie horizontal, making it difficult for small children to breathe thoracically; they persist with diaphragmatic movement. If these children suffer pain in the abdomen they may develop chest infections as they find their breathing movements compromised.

Changes in posture are related to development of the secondary spinal curves. At four months babies pull their heads up and try to

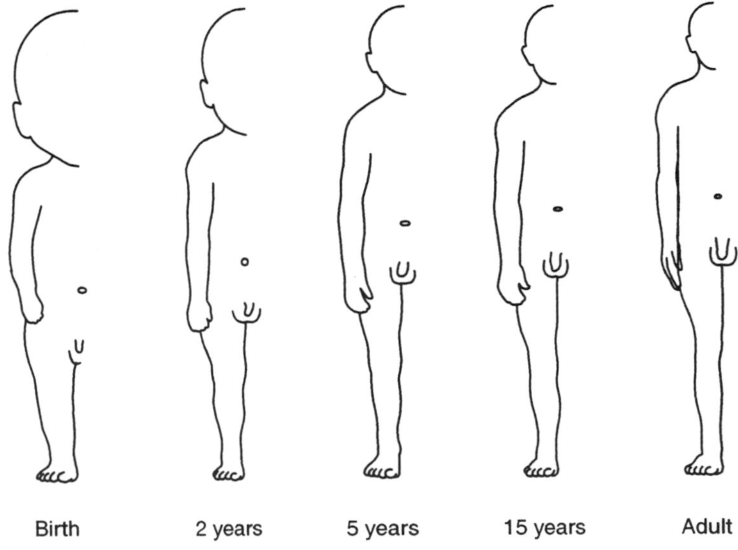

Figure 2.5 How body proportions change with age

balance the head on top of the spine to fix gaze. At eight months they have the muscle strength to sit up, and the lumbar curve appears. At one year, standing against gravity needs a wide gait to balance the heavy skull, and the lumbar curve may be exaggerated, with abdomen protruding, in order to hold the upper part of the body erect until the back muscles develop the strength to maintain posture.

In the adolescent spurt the feet and hands grow first, then the calf and forearm, hips and chest, then the shoulders. Adolescent children are often accused of being clumsy; however, their bodies may have grown at such a rate that their brains have not yet reorganised spatially. The bones of the face grow, sinuses develop and the jaw drops down. Permanent teeth erupt as the 'ugly ducking' evolves. When the sex hormones take effect on the skeleton in puberty, boys' shoulders develop in response to use of their stronger pectoral muscles. In girls the pelvis becomes wider and shallower, and body fat deposits occur; the girl's shape may affect other parts of the skeleton to produce 'knock knees', flat feet and a curved thoracic spine. Towards the end of this rapid spurt the child begins to grow laterally and 'fill out'. Sheldon's three different components of physique or somatotypes – endomorph, mesomorph and ectomorph – can be recognised by the age of twenty years. These are part influenced by genetic inheritance and part by the effect of individual physical activity habit and hormone influence.

All these body changes have a profound affect on each individual's psychological response throughout their childhood. Toddlers who can jump in puddles will experience mastery over their world; eight-year-olds who can ride a bike will experience the thrill of attaining a skill; the young person who sees an adult body emerging will need to constantly reshape his or her identity. Physical change will also determine new social roles and expectations, and children who are too small or too big compared to their peer group will experience advantages and disadvantages in equal measure. All these body changes have profound affects on each individual's psychological wellbeing.

Physiology knowledge in practice

Scenario 1

You are visiting a Muslim family who have recently arrived in the UK with their baby son and five-year-old daughter. What are the main areas of information, in relation to healthy bones, that you would expect to hear from the health visitor when giving routine advice to this mother?

Some pointers:

- Children need fresh air, sunlight, a balanced diet and exercise in order that their skeletons grow strong.
- The children would benefit from being taken out each day to the local park to walk and play. It would increase their exposure to their new environment and give them interests to stimulate their learning. Oxygen in the air is needed by osteoblasts and osteoclasts for the release of energy to break down, remove and build new bone tissue; they can get this in the home but there will more space for them to be active in the outside areas.
- Mum will have to ensure that the children's skins are exposed to ultraviolet radiation to encourage epidermal cells in the stratum spinosum and stratum germinativum to convert a steroid related to cholesterol into vitamin D. In a country where the sunlight is strong and more frequently seen, the culture is to avoid its rays and cover skin to protect it. Vitamin D is vital to bone development and is absorbed, modified and released by the liver and then converted by the kidneys into calcitriol, which is needed for the absorption of calcium and phosphorus by the small intestine (Thibodeau and Patton 2007).
- Mum will have to adjust her use of ingredients for the family diet as some of these may not be immediately accessible near her new home. Calcium is important for all of them but more so for the children whose bones are growing. It gives the skeleton its strength. It is a mineral found in milk and other dairy products and bony fish; the professional will have to discuss alternatives in relation to the preferred family requirements. Mum may still be breastfeeding her baby and the health visitor will need to advise her on her diet to sustain this and suitable weaning foods available to her son. Vitamin D, not so available from sunlight activity on subcutaneous fat in the winter months in the UK, can be found in fatty foods such as margarine, butter and red meat. The health visitor will have to discuss the change of diet for the family and ensure this mineral and vitamin is available for them in foods they enjoy and are familiar with.

- Exercise that is weight bearing puts stress on to the epiphyseal plates of the long bones, which encourages osteoclasts to lay down mineral in the bone cartilage matrix. The five-year-old girl should be encouraged to take part in a range of activities that includes climbing, running and jumping and walking to school and the baby should be helped to sit, crawl and eventually walk through play interaction. A local mother and child group would help support this mother, especially if there were a mixture of new immigrants integrating into the UK society and child care sessions were part of the ongoing programme.

Scenario 2

Jane, aged nine years, has been referred to the school nurse by her teacher because she seems to have become lethargic and reluctant to take part in physical activities during school time. The school nurse finds that Jane spends all her time at home watching TV and has a very restricted self imposed diet. She appears depressed after her parents' divorce. This is a complicated case, but why should Jane need intervention in relation to her skeletal development?

The theory (Rodriguez 2006):

- Jane needs to eat properly and take part in the school's physical activity programme for her future health.
- Jane is at the stage of her development when she is growing fast under the stimulus of her sex hormones. This period of rapid growth is stimulated by gonadotrophin secretion. Her skeleton is getting bigger and bone is being deposited at the epiphiseal plates in direct relation to her activity levels. Bone growth is an increase in osteocyte numbers, and intracellular substance – the bone matrix.
- Three hours of sport each week, such as netball or gymnastics, induces a peak bone mass in the adult status; weight bearing generates compromise forces on the growth plates. Intensity is more important than duration to build this strength, thus tensile, compressive, shear, bending and torsion stress have the osteogenic potential.
- Sport also increases lean muscle mass, especially skeletal muscle mass, which is a predictor of bone mineral mass accrual, as it

will increase the tension on bone to deposit calcium. Sport activities before puberty leads to bigger bones, increased ossification of the lumbar spine and a femoral bone mass which lasts for life. In the two-year period of the growth spurt at eleven to thirteen years in females (twelve to fourteen years in males), 25 per cent of total adult bone mass is attained.

- Lean muscle mass and fat accumulation precedes this bone mass development. Jane must keep her body weight within a normal range for her height and be encouraged to become more active within the school day.

Extend your knowledge

Read 'Contribution of timetabled physical education to total physical activity in primary school children', Mallan *et al.*'s 2003 article, and do your own research activity! Ask children you work with what physical activities they enjoy and how often they take part in them. Then watch the children in your care and observe how active they are/are not at play. Mallan *et al.* measured the extent of children's effort in physical activity. You might like to consider this as you watch different individuals taking part in both structured and unstructured physical activity and whether they make more effort if the activity is what they chose to do.

? Quiz

1 Name the two types of bone cell.

2 Where are the primary ossification centres?

3 What are the four spinal curves and which one develops first?

4 Describe the resuscitation position of the head for a child of four years and why this knowledge is needed for safe practice.

5 Suggest four things that affect skeletal growth – other than Growth Hormone (GH).

6 Explain the 'Christmas tree effect' in children's growth.

7 GH is activated by what intermediate chemical and where is it produced?

8 What is a chalone?

9 What affect does GH have on blood proteins, fats, minerals and glucose?

10 Explain how calcitonin antogonises parathyroid hormone.

11 Cortisol is a stress hormone – explain its effect on bone tissue.

12 In what way do androgens affect the female development?

13 What hormones antagonise insulin?

14 How does oestrogen aid bone growth?

15 Why do boys have a heavier skeleton and stronger muscles than girls?

16 At what age do children need the most calcium in their diet?

17 Physical activity increases bone mass – what activities are best for children?

18 Why are some children physically stronger than others?

19 Why might a teenager be considered 'clumsy'?

20 Explain how normal physical growth might increase a child's self-esteem.

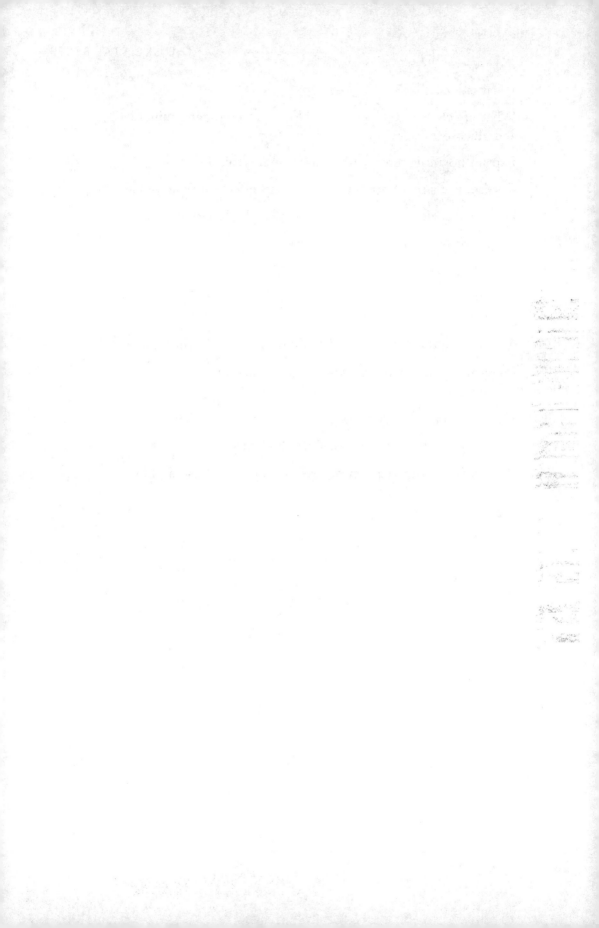

Chapter 3

The nervous system

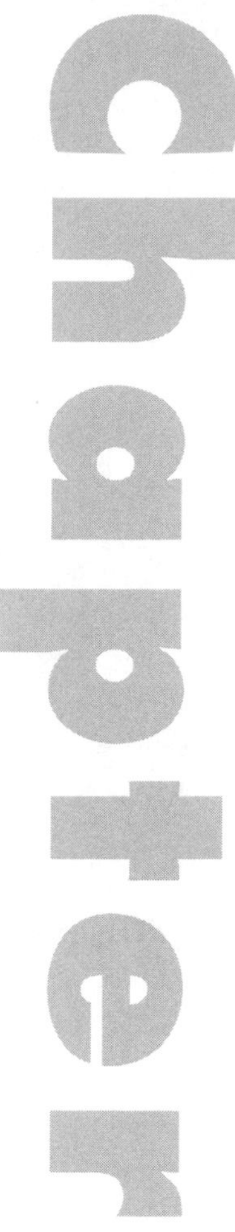

- Brain growth embryology
- Temperature control
- Nerve growth
- The blood/brain barrier
- Birth and the primitive reflexes
- Sensory nerve function
- Neuromuscular control
- Sleep

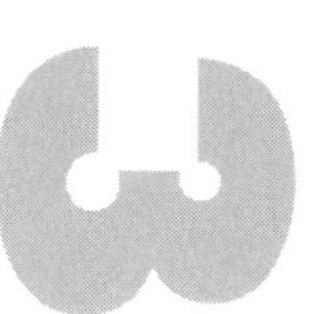

BRAIN DEVELOPMENT occurs at several stages during childhood. The critical period for brain growth appears to be during the first sixteen weeks of life. At birth, a baby's brain weighs approximately 25 per cent of its future adult weight. By the time the child is two years old the brain has increased to 75 per cent, and by six years, 90 per cent of its eventual weight. This, then, indicates phenomenal growth of the central nervous system during the early years. Peripheral nerves continue to become myelinated (grow fatty sheaths to increase nerve transmission rate) and fine physical control appears as the child moves towards adult status. With the unique environment impinging on every waking and sleeping hour, this plastic nervous system constantly matures and changes as demands are put upon it. The nervous system coordinates and controls all body systems to a greater or lesser degree and, together with the hormones of the endocrine system, fine-tunes a delicate homeostasis.

Brain growth embryology

The brain starts its development soon after conception; it is vulnerable to damage through pregnancy. The first indication of the nervous system is within the neural plate, a thickened area of the ectoderm that forms after the ovum has been fertilised in the third week of gestation, and by the end of this week the neural folds have begun to fuse to the median plane to form the neural tube. This neural tube is the beginning of the brain and spinal cord. As the neural tube separates from the surface ectoderm cells, the neural folds form the neural crest. Ganglia of the spine, cranial and autonomic nervous system develop from the neural crest. The embryo at twenty-three days shows the hindbrain and midbrain to be formed, and the neural tube closes. In the fourth week the head folds begin to develop as the forebrain grows rapidly. In the fifth week the eye starts to grow, and cerebral hemispheres also develop from this area. The nerves of the branchial arches become the cranial nerves. Peak head breadth growth velocity occurs at thirteen post-menstrual weeks, although a relatively high velocity continues to about thirty weeks. Peak head circumference velocity occurs two to three weeks later, because the cerebellum situated at the back of the skull grows later than the cerebrum. Head volume, representing brain size, has its peak velocity at thirty weeks and growth rapidly slows after this. Different parts

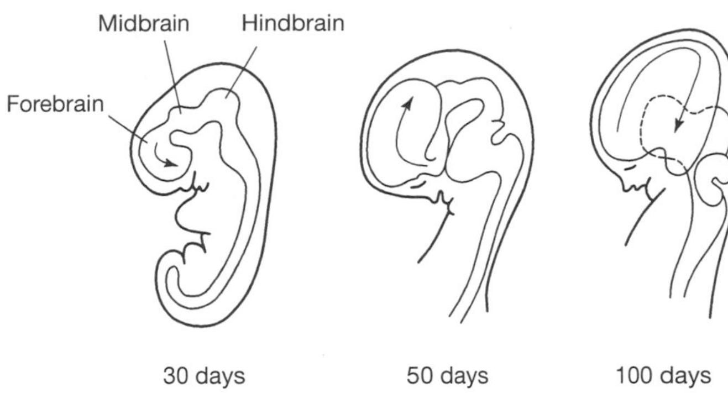

Figure 3.1 Brain growth – thirty to one hundred days

of the brain grow at different rates, but the hindbrain and midbrain remain the most advanced.

The two hemispheres of the human brain are not mirror images of each other; the upper surface of the temporal lobe and the whole occipital region is larger on the left side than on the right. The perception functions of the left brain are more specialised for the analysis of stimuli sequences which occur one after the other whereas the right brain analyses space, shape and form which are presented at the same time. The right hemisphere processes spatial information, both visual and tactile. There is some debate as to how the sex hormones affect brain development in relation to gender identity. Bee and Boyd (2007) offer a debate on gender and sex and how children develop the coherent sense of 'self'. One part of the frontal lobe on the left side is called Broca's area; this is where muscle movements are controlled for the mouth and lips and thus speech production. It communicates closely with a superior part of the temporal lobe called Wernicke's area where speech production is coordinated. Speech comprehension begins in the auditory system and is comprehended and translated to words in the left side of the brain in Wernicke's area. Reading is related to listening and talking ability and children's brains have usually matured for this complex activity by the age of five years (see Figure 3.1).

In the newborn, the brain is 10 to 12 per cent of body weight, weighs approximately 450 grams and is 25 per cent of the adult size. It doubles in the first year of life, growth spurts occurring at one-month intervals for the first five months and then at eight, twelve and twenty months. Between the ages of two and four years brain growth slows and then shows another major spurt at four years. Bee and Boyd explain how the growth spurts in the brain are correlated to cognitive milestones, such as the development of language fluency in the fourth year and the increase in size of the temporal lobe, and in the teenage years qualitative changes in the neural network allow the young person to think more abstractly. Nerve connections and their networks are, however, dependent on day to day experiences to establish 'attunement'; a more complex network of nerve connections. How the child responds to stimuli in their early life allows them to adapt their responses and is reliant on rich stimulation for optimal development.

To accommodate this growth the sutures between the skull bones are not yet fused at birth, and there are two openings in the skull which can be easily felt. The anterior fontanelle, which can be felt in the midline of the skull above the brow, closes gradually in the first eighteen months of life, while the smaller posterior fontanelle, again in the midline but towards the back of the baby's head, is normally closed by the age of six weeks. The anterior fontanelle is normally flat when palpated but may pulsate with the heartbeat or bulge when the baby coughs or strains. It may feel soft or slightly springy from the support of the layer of the cerebral spinal fluid, which circulates under the arachnoid membrane to cushion and protect the delicate brain. If the fontanelle appears depressed the child may be dehydrated. If it bulges it may indicate that the flow of cerebral spinal fluid is impeded, such as in the child with hydrocephalus or meningitis.

The brain volume is reflected in head circumference measured at the greatest circumference from the top of the eyebrows and pinna of the ears to the occipital prominence of the skull. The head circumference increases by 8–9 cm in the first year of life. It is an important measurement of brain development. Good practice requires the measurement to be of the greatest circumference which is slightly above the eyebrows and pinna of the ears and around the occipital prominence at the back of the skull (Glasper *et al.* 2007).

The most active parts of the brain at birth (see Figure 3.2) are the sensorimotor cortex, the thalamus, the brain stem and the cerebellum. All the major surface features of the cerebral hemispheres are present at birth, but the cerebral cortex is only half its adult thickness. The spinal cord is about 15–18 cm long, with its lower end opposite either the second or third lumbar vertebra. The spinal cord does not grow as much as the vertebral canal and therefore

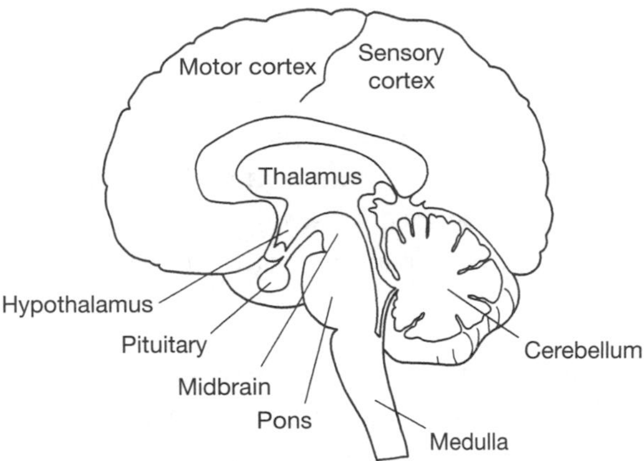

Figure 3.2 The most active parts of the brain at birth

appears to rise up as the child grows in length. All the major sensory tracts are fairly well myelinated, but the motor tracts less so. However, the local reflexes related to swallowing and sucking appear before birth and have their nerve pathways well myelinated.

Temperature control

Temperature control in children is not completed until approximately five years of age; this may be due to the immaturity of the nervous system and the tissues it services. The maintenance of body temperature is mainly coordinated by the hypothalamus, a vital central control centre containing large numbers of heat-sensitive neurones called thermoreceptors. It is an important homeostatic mechanism which allows the body enzymes to work efficiently within a narrow range of 32–42 °C. In response to a change in temperature, the peripheral thermoreceptors transmit signals to the hypothalamus, where they are integrated with the receptor signals from the preoptic area of the brain.

Heat is created by:

- metabolism in the liver, skeletal muscles and other chemical actions. Metabolism releases chemical energy from the covalent bonds of hydrogen compounds, fat and carbohydrates, and the energy that is not used for cell activity is lost as heat;

- shivering, the involuntary spasmotic contraction and relaxation of skeletal muscles creating heat by muscle work, which occurs when the environmental or core temperatures drop;
- the pilomotor reflex, which makes hair on the skin stand up due to contraction of the pilomotor muscles in the hair follicles, insulating the skin surface by stopping the convection of cooler air that takes away heat from the body surface (Marieb and Hoehn 2007).

When babies are placed in a cool environment, metabolic activities occur that can result in hypoglycaemia, elevated serum bilirubin, metabolic acidosis and increased metabolic rate. When heat loss begins, non-shivering thermogenesis (NST) heat production is triggered by thermoreceptors in the subcutaneous tissue, hypothalamus and spinal cord.

This heat production may begin within the first four hours after birth from the 'cold stress' of delivery because the forty-week gestation (normal term) baby has a certain amount of 'brown fat'. This accounts for 4 per cent of their total fat mass and is found around the kidney and adrenal muscles and blood vessels of the neck, in the mediastinum and the scapular and axillae. Brown fat is deposited between weeks twenty-six to thirty of gestation but is insufficient in quantity to be useful until week thirty-six. Thus, very premature babies are not able to generate much heat for themselves and are usually cared for in warmed incubators. Brown fat metabolism triggers fat breakdown to generate heat. Blood vessel dilation from this local heat production then results in 25 per cent of the cardiac output flowing through these dilated vessels to maintain core temperature. During this process oxygen is used by brown fat at three times the rate of other body tissues and can result in a metabolic acidosis which will compete with bilirubin for blood albumin sites, and thus the bilirubin levels will rise. At birth, the foetal haemoglobin is broken down rapidly and bilirubin levels normally increase, thus if blood albumen is not available to remove it, jaundice can develop if the baby is allowed to become cold.

Glucose is also used at a higher rate by brown fat; if replacement of energy from food is not addressed, the infant will eventually become hypo-glycaemic and convulse as the brain becomes deprived of sugar.

In measuring temperature by axilla in the term baby, one may assume it is warm whereas the infant is, perhaps, too cold. It is recommended to take both tympanic (core) and axilla (shell) temperature in the infant if the professional is in doubt.

Heat is lost:

- through contact with a cooler environment;
- by vasodilation, where the peripheral blood vessels dilate due to inhibition of the sympathetic centres in the posterior hypothalamus;
- by sweating, where the preoptic area in the anterior hypothalamus is stimulated causing secretion of water to the skin surface for evaporation;
- by a decrease in heat-producing activity (Edwards 1998).

Thus, in measuring temperature in children it is important to clarify the observed characteristics of changes from normal. The immature brain has a more labile homeostatic control than the adult. Under five years of age, children's brains become irritated by overheating. Parents and carers may observe changes in skin colour, posture, fluid intake and output, and level of activity and behaviour (A.J.S. Brown, cited in Glasper *et al.* 2007, feverish illness at www.nice.org.uk). However, as temperature has a circadian rhythm, a reading of 37.5 °C at 14.00 hours will not necessarily indicate a fever, but taken at 02.00 hours it may. Normal temperature of an infant at night may be 36.0 °C and rise to 37.8 °C if active in the day, giving a normal mean of 36.9 °C (Casey 2000).

There are many tools on the market today to measure temperature:

- The tympanic membrane infrared device is favoured in hospitals as it is quick to use and reflects the blood passing through the ear and servicing the hypothalamus, thus giving a core reading. However, it is expensive and the earpiece needs to be the correct size for the size of the child. It is not accurate if the eardrum is occluded by cerumen or a disease state, such as an inflammation of the tympanic membrane (A.J.S. Brown, cited in Glasper *et al.* 2007).
- An axilla reading taken with an electronic probe is easy to access and safe, but can give a false reading if the child is sweating or has a large layer of insulating fat. A small child can squirm and dislodge this type of probe from the skin surface.
- The mercury/glass clinical thermometer used in the mouth is not considered safe for many children, as they cannot hold it

correctly with the mercury reservoir under the tongue near the lingual artery.

- Disposable thermometers are popular with families as they pose no safety threat, are reasonably accurate and are easily available from the high street pharmacy.

Nerve growth

The principal cells of the brain are neurones. They have long processes of two types: the single axon and one or more shorter dendrites. These neurones are the cells that carry messages throughout the body, and they occupy half of the brain volume. The neurones are supported by a group of cells called neuroglia, which provide nutrition and defence and repair of the neurons:

- Oligodendrocytes are responsible for myelination of axons in the central nervous system. They can myelinate several processes at any one time (see Figure 3.3). These neuroglia migrate to the axons or nerve fibres of the nerve cells throughout childhood, wrap themselves round the long nerve extensions and develop fatty cylinders which insulate the nerve fibres. These fatty sheaths allow the passage of nerve impulses to speed up and thus produce effects more quickly. The quicker nerve impulses allow the child

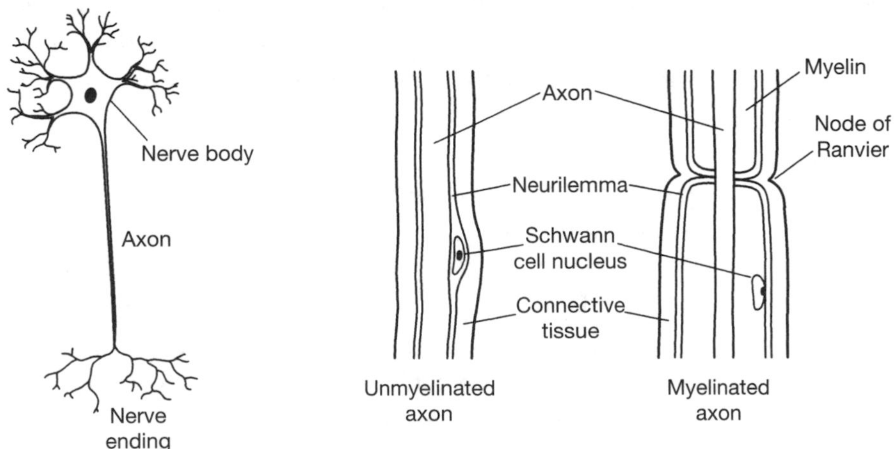

Figure 3.3 Axon myelination

to become more accurate with all physical activities such as hand writing and riding a bicycle.

- Schwann cells ensheath the axons of peripheral nerve axons. Their myeline sheath of 80 per cent lipids and 20 per cent protein insulates the nerve axon and allows rapid transmission of nerve impulse. Myelination of the nerve axons is a process that continues after birth. The nodes of Ranvier, spaces between the Schwann cells, appear constant as the nerve axon grows. As the internodal spaces elongate, the speed of transmission of the nerve impulse increases. In general, the thicker the nerve the thicker the myeline sheath that wraps around it.
- Satellite cells encapsulate dorsal root and cranial nerve ganglion cells and regulate their micro-environment.
- Astrocytes occupy interneurone spaces and connect to small blood vessels, thus allowing neurone nutrition. Their processes surround groups of synaptic endings in the central nervous system and isolate them from adjacent synapses. Their foot processes connect the blood vessels with the connective tissue at the surface of the central nervous system, which may help limit the free diffusion of substances into the central nervous system itself.
- Microglia transform to phagocytes when cells in the nervous system are damaged, and are probably derived from the circulation.
- Ependymal cells line the ventricles of the brain and separate the chambers for the central nervous system tissue. Many substances diffuse easily across them between the extracellular space of the brain and the cerebral spinal fluid.

Growth in nerve cell size occurs as the early embryonic neurones absorb nutrients and fluids from their environment. Once formed, a nerve cell can increase in mass up to 200,000 times, most of the addition being to the processes of the cells. Each of these processes may come to contain as much as a thousand times the amount of material contained in the cell body. The diameter of the myelinated nerve cells in peripheral nerve trunks increases considerably; the nerve cells contain much RNA (ribonucleic acid), which is used to form cytoplasm to be pushed into rapidly growing dendrites. By eighteen weeks' gestation, most of the neurons' nuclei are formed in the cerebrum, but neuroglial cells continue to be produced here up to two years of age. Neuroglial cells in the cerebellum, on the other hand, begin to form earlier at fifteen weeks and continue to be formed until fifteen months after birth. By six months' gestation, nerve cells are growing in size rather than dividing, and there is a huge increase in the cytoplasm that allows interconnections, ramification and myelination of their processes to occur.

The blood/brain barrier

The blood/brain barrier is an anatomical/physiological feature of the brain that separates brain parenchyma from blood. It is formed chiefly by tight junctions between capillary endothelial cells of the blood vessels. These cerebral capillaries have no fenestrations or pores, and are thought to be responsible for the selective nature of the blood/ brain barrier when mature. The blood/brain barrier is a term used to describe its function, based on observations that facilitated diffusion of glucose. Essential amino acids, some electrolytes and passive diffusion of water and carbon dioxide is allowed, but it is impermeable to non essential amino acids and potassium ions. Histological evidence shows astrocyte processes, capillary endothelium and neurone membranes to be closely associated and their cell membranes to contain potassium pumps (Bear *et al.* 2007). The brain is ineffective against fats, fatty acids and other fat soluble substances such as alcohol, nicotine and anaesthetics (Marieb and Hoehn 2007). However, in the foetus and newborn, it is indiscriminately permeable, allowing passage of protein and other large and small molecules to pass freely between the cerebral vessels and the brain. Harmful substances such as lead have been found to accumulate in certain individuals exposed to this metal; but most ions such as sodium and potassium are regulated in order not to disrupt the transmission of nerve impulses. The blood/brain barrier functions to exclude substances that are of low solubility in lipid, such as organic acids, highly ionised polar compounds, large molecules and substances not transported by specific carrier-mediated transport systems. These include albumin and substances bound to albumin such as bilirubin, many hormones and drugs, organic and inorganic toxins. Because the young child does not have mature function, osmotic changes and free bilirubin in the blood, for example, will allow water and bilirubin to enter and damage brain tissue in abnormal circumstances (Marieb and Hoehn 2007). Conditions that cause cerebrovascular dilation, such as hypertension, hypercapnia, hypoxia and acidosis, disrupt the blood/brain barrier.

Hyperosmotic fluids which cause shrinkage of vascular endothelium, and thus widen the vascular junctions, also interfere with normal protective function.

Birth and the primitive reflexes

Young babies at birth are equipped with a number of primitive instinctive movements which assist their survival. These motor responses are extensions of those established during foetal life. These patterns take the form of reflexes that are either present at birth or appear in infancy. Some of the reflexes are simple and are mediated at the spinal cord level; others are more complex and require the integration of brain centres, the labyrinths and other developing nervous centres.

The new baby can:

- blink – the corneal and blinking reflexes are strong and can be seen when the baby is carried in a draught or faced towards the sun;
- yawn, cough, sneeze, defecate and micturate, taste and smell, and withdraw from pain;
- cry, root, suck and swallow – these primitive reflexes associated with feeding, the tongue retrusion reflex, are well developed at birth;
- grasp a finger if placed in the palm of the hand – this palmar grasp is a flexor response and is characterised by a relatively strong flexion of the palm and fingers without thumb opposition and will curl the foot if the plantar surface is equally stroked (Babinski sign);
- show a Moro sign if their position is quickly changed. The Moro reflex, where the startled child will fling his or her arms symmetrically apart and then bring them together again, is the most consistent primitive developmental milestone between birth and three months. The extensor response can be demonstrated by any sudden movement of the neck region. The infant reacts with extension and abduction of the extremities and a noticeable tremor of the hands and feet;
- show the startle reflex – similar to the Moro and is stimulated by a loud unexpected noise; the baby responds as with the

> Moro response but with flexion rather than abduction of the extremities.
>
> (London *et al.* 2006)

A second set of reflexes, the locomotor reflexes, resemble later voluntary movements that will allow the child to move through space. These include creeping, standing, stepping and swimming. They can show many body movements such as prone crawling and turning the pelvis to a stroking stimulus of the spine (Galant sign). They can show a stepping reflex if feet are suspended against a table edge. One can elicit a response to move their eyes to fix on a face by stroking the cheek so they turn their heads towards this stimulus. Many children also find this stroking activity comforting when distressed (Moyse 2005). These movements do not involve voluntary control at first, and indicate a lack of inhibition of the segmental apparatus of the nervous system. As this matures in infancy and childhood, the inhibitory functions of the cerebral cortex begin to operate, and these reflex movements gradually diminish and are integrated into voluntary patterns. There is much variation in these reflex responses in children as well as within the same child – they may change with behavioural states. However, their presence or absence is indicative of normal nervous system development and vital to later ability to walk, run and jump.

The third group of reflexes in the newborn are the postural reflexes. One of these is the tonic neck reflex. This develops in the first few months of life. When the baby's head is turned to one side it responds with an increased muscle tone and extension of both the arm and the leg of the side to which the face is turned, and by the flexion of the arm and leg of the opposite side. Another postural reflex, the righting reflex, facilitates maintenance of the relationship between the head and other body parts. The third postural reflex, the labyrinthine reflex, orientates the body relative to the force of gravity. These postural reflexes begin to emerge at about three months and increase in intensity throughout infancy. Their function is to help the baby maintain or regain its balance against gravity when disturbed.

It appears that the primitive reflexes disappear as functional abilities, such as turning towards sound, gazing at moving objects, reaching under conscious control for attractive objects, increased manipulative control and weight bearing through legs, allow mobility to develop (Bee and Boyd 2007).

The new baby faces two main challenges in development: to learn about its environment and to stand upright against gravity. The first neurological assessment, soon after birth, is a good indicator of body function and uses the Apgar score where normal, poor and absent are given points from two to zero. A total score below 7 indicates moderate neuromuscular/cardiorespiratory depression and needs monitoring. The five components of this assessment are heart rate, respiratory effort, muscle tone, response to stimuli and colour.

Sensory nerve function

Skin

In the peripheral skin there are marked changes in the neural pattern. During the third month of intrauterine life the epidermis begins to stratify, and is immediately invaded by branches from the cutaneous plexus of nerves. As the organised endings appear in the skin, the intraepidermal fibres and endings withdraw, so that after birth only a few remain. In the dermis the organised sensory endings, such as the Meissner corpuscles, are closely packed together but as the skin grows they become thinned out. Thus, the tiny baby has acute skin sensation, but as the child grows the skin receptors become more differentially and widely spaced particularly over the dorsal surface of the body but more concentrated in areas such as the breast and inner thigh where skin remains more sensitive to touch.

Touch can be a calming communication with children; peripheral nerve endings are stimulated through the autonomic nervous system. Pulse rate, respiration rate, oxygen consumption, blood pressure and muscle tension are lowered, gut motility, peripheral flow and white blood cells production are enhanced (London *et al.* 2006). Massage can be beneficial to both communicating and supporting the physical health of the young. The newborn's skin is very thin and the epidermis is loosely bound to the dermis; friction can cause blisters.

Sweat is speedily produced in response to temperature rise and emotion. The apocrine glands are small and the oil production is non-functioning; good practice advises that infants need bathing infrequently and then not in water containing soap products which will further dry their fragile skin. There is less melanin available for protection against sunlight; young children should not be exposed to intensive sunlight for long periods.

As the child moves into adolescence the epidermis thickens and binds with the dermis so there is better protection against infection and external trauma. Both boys and girls produce oil on the skin; these glands are activated by the androgens of the adrenal cortex. The control of overactive sebaceous glands and infections in acne cause difficulty for the emerging adult. Boys produce more sweat than girls because of the higher muscle mass and heat production, but both become better protected from the sun as melanin production achieves mature function.

The eye

The neural parts of the eye are evident at the fourth week after conception, when optic grooves develop in the neural folds at the cranial end of the embryo. The optic nerve and lens is present at seven weeks and the eyelids develop from the folds of the surface ectoderm and fuse at the eighth week of foetal life. The lacrimal gland develops at ten weeks. The eyes remain closed until about week twenty-eight of gestation (London *et al.* 2006).

The cells of the visual area of the cortex have their peak burst of development in the period between twenty-eight and thirty-two weeks' gestation. The 'visual analyser' starts to myelinate shortly before birth and completes rapidly by the tenth week after birth to cope with visual stimuli. The cornea and lens of the eye cast an image of the environment on the photoreceptors of the retina, each of which will respond to the intensity of the light that falls on it. A mosaic pattern is formed which passes via the optic nerves, optic chiasma and thalamus to the visual cortex in the occipital lobe of the cerebrum. Several other regions of the brain, including the hypothalamus and brain stem, will also receive visual information. These other regions help regulate activity during the day/night cycle, coordinate eye and head movements, control attention to visual stimuli and regulate the size of the pupils (Carlson 2001). Some mothers report their baby to have a day/night cycle in the third trimester of pregnancy; perhaps the light-sensitive retina begins to signal a light/dark rhythm at this time.

Harris and Butterworth (2002) report that very young babies see the normal colour range of blue, green, yellow and red, but children need to focus light on to the central part of the retina, the fovea, for the colour receptors, known as cones, to develop. There seems to be a critical time for development of the fovea, which is about the age of three to four years. After this age surgical correction of strabismus, a common reason for light not being focused correctly to the retina, will not produce optimal function. The eyeball is at first too short for its lens, so most infants have about one dioptre of long sightedness. As it grows, the eyeball becomes longer but the converging power of the cornea and lens reduces, thus cancelling out the refractive error of the newborn. Stereoscopic vision develops at thirteen weeks when the eye muscles allow eyes to converge on an object. One needs to hold small babies at a distance of about 20 cm when talking to them as the lens at this age does not accommodate, but by six months they can focus on the feeding bottle and recognise their parent from across a room. The lens then continues to grow throughout life; at fourteen years it is of adult size, but by sixty years it is one-third bigger than the young adult of twenty years.

The ear

The outer ear, the auricle, grows at the same rate as the body developing from the dorsal portion of the branchial groove. The inner ear develops as an otic pit either side of the hindbrain early in the fourth week after conception, and is complete by the eighth week of embryonic life. The middle ear develops from the first pharyngeal pouch and soon envelopes the middle ear bones which develop from the first and second branchial arches. The fibres of the 'acoustic analyser' (Carlson 2001) begin to myelinate at the sixth month of foetal life but do not complete until the end of the fourth year, possibly in relation to the development of language.

In the womb babies are sensitive to sounds from their mothers' viscera, the foetus can hear at twenty weeks gestation. Sound waves are transmitted to the inner ear, and via the auditory nerve to the medulla; the inner ear controls posture, head movement and eye movement. Information received in the medulla relays it to the cerebellum, spinal cord, pons and temporal cortex. Neurones also synapse here to the auditory cortex in the temporal lobe, with the stimulus mainly going to the same hemisphere as the ear receiving the sound. Newborn babies can detect pitch, loudness and timbre of sound, and also location and changes in complex sounds. They appear well programmed to listen to their mothers' voice and be soothed by this sound.

The inner ear, the middle ear cavity and the drum (tympanic membrane) are fully formed at eight weeks' gestation and of almost adult size at birth. Sound waves move air molecules, focused by the pinna to the external meatus, that impact on the tympanic membrane at the end of the passage from the outer ear. This membrane vibrates and moves the three bones of the middle ear which, in turn, vibrate against the inner ear membrane, a communication window to the fluid filled cochlea. In the cochlea the fluid waves disrupt fine hairs that stimulate the auditory nerve. The auditory nerve then transmits a nerve impulse to the temporal lobe for interpretation by the cerebral cortex of the brain. Hearing is a complex activity that relies on a sophisticated and coordinated pathway of physiological function. The difference between a child's and adult's ear is that the Eustachian tube is wider and shorter and the meatus is straighter from the pinna to the tympanic membrane. Thus, children are more susceptible to middle ear deafness from throat infections ascending the Eustachian tube than adults because of this difference in anatomy; they also are prone to inserting small objects into this orifice such as peas and beads! Grommets are commonly inserted to 'air' the middle ear in children under the age of eight years. These small tubes allow the three oscillating bones to conduct sound waves to the inner ear and allow auditory nerve stimulation. Poor hearing will impede the acquisition of language.

Beginnings of language development

Coordination and maturation of neural responses, especially those of mouth articulation, sight, hearing and cognition, are vital for the development of language in any part of the world. Early reflexes mature in a stimulating environment to allow the child to interact meaningfully and make sense of their world. A constant interaction with a carer facilitates this process; talking to children gives them the experiences and practice of oral communication and the foundation for organising their thoughts, expressing themselves and preparing them for reading and writing skills.

Noises made from birth to two months are a reflexive vocalisation of sounds to express discomfort and distress and relates to bodily functions. The quality of the expressed sounds changes at two to four months when the baby can respond to communication by cooing and laughing. At three months the larynx is high, so the epiglottis nearly touches the soft palate at the back of the mouth. The tongue is large in relation to the size of the mouth, the pharynx is short; this back part of the tongue cannot be manipulated. However, it is ideal for sucking. At four to six months the production of more sophisticated sound increases in vocal play where the child gains control of articulation of the larynx and mouth and experiments in loudness, pitch and the position of the tongue. Children of this age love to play games that require them to practise this skill, sometimes inappropriately at meal times. From three to nine months there is increasing control of fine movements and a range of sounds such as da, ba, wa, de, ha, he appear in all languages. By seven or eight months babies begin to show understanding of familiar words in relation to their experience of them (Harris and Butterworth 2002).

Motor nerve function

At birth much of the nerve tissue still has little myeline insulation; thus the rate of nerve transmission is slower than in the adult and the movement is less efficient. This control of movement improves as the myeline increases and the child interacts with the environment. Although there is a wide range of normal movements, the sequence of development shows the same steps. First is the cephalocaudal, or head-to-toe development, as the child shows the ability to control the head and face before the lower limbs. Development is also proximodistal where the development of the midline occurs before that of the extremities; the baby controls the arm before the fingers. The child controls the general before the specific; the arm-waving motion is gained before the finer control of manipulating a toy. At all ages balance and the ability to control the head, trunk and limbs is important; later the gait and the ability to control the body in space is a necessary milestone. A baby's level of consciousness can be assessed by its level of activity and interest in the environment and its interaction with people. The baby's motor development reflects the neuromuscular maturation and is related to the rapid growth of the brain at this time. The association, noticeable in the infant stage, may be related to the unique growth spurt of the cerebellum. This controls the development and maintenance of neuromuscular coordination, balance and muscle tone. Whereas in the rest of the brain there is a spurt in the number of neuroglial cells, the cerebellum starts its spurt later than the cerebrum and brain stem but completes it earlier. The cerebrum and brain stem begin their growth spurt at about mid-pregnancy, whereas the cerebellum starts a month or two before term. By eighteen months of age the estimated cell count of the cerebellum has reached adult levels, whereas the cerebrum and brain stem have achieved only 60 per cent. It is during this time that the infant develops the postural control and balance needed for walking.

Neuromuscular control

Two clear gradients occur in the cerebral cortex during the first two years after birth: the first to do with general functional areas (see Figure 3.4) and the second to do with body location.

There are three general functional areas. The most advanced part of the cortex is the primary motor area located in the pre-central gyrus, the cells which initiate movement. The second area to develop is the primary sensory area in the post-central gyrus where nerve fibres mediate the sense of touch. The third area to develop is the primary visual area in the occipital lobe where nerve paths from the retina end.

Body locomotion

In the motor area control of arm and upper trunk develops ahead of those controlling the leg which can take at least two years to

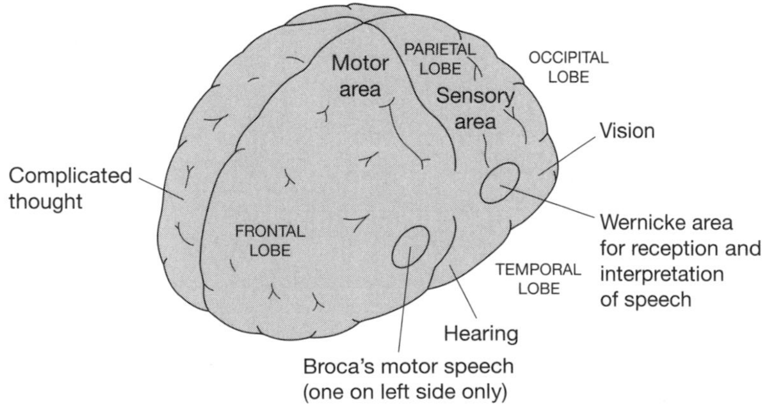

Figure 3.4 General functional areas in the cerebral cortex

develop fully. A number of motor tracts will not have completed their myelination even after four years of life. During the first two years of life the child gradually attains postural, locomotor and prehensile control (Figure 3.5). Motor development is viewed as representing neuromuscular maturation; gross motor skills which develop earlier at all ages, such as crawling and walking, and fine motor skills which develop later, such as holding a pencil. However, motor development is a plastic process, and variation in the sequence, timing and rate of development is most likely to relate to a variety of biological (genetic, body size and composition) and environmental (rearing atmosphere, play opportunities and objects) factors.

Walking is a major task for the two-year-old. There has to be prior control of the head, upper trunk and upper limbs, then the control of the entire trunk, in the development of sitting unaided. Creeping and crawling is then followed by standing with and without support. This advanced ability is usually achieved by fifteen months.

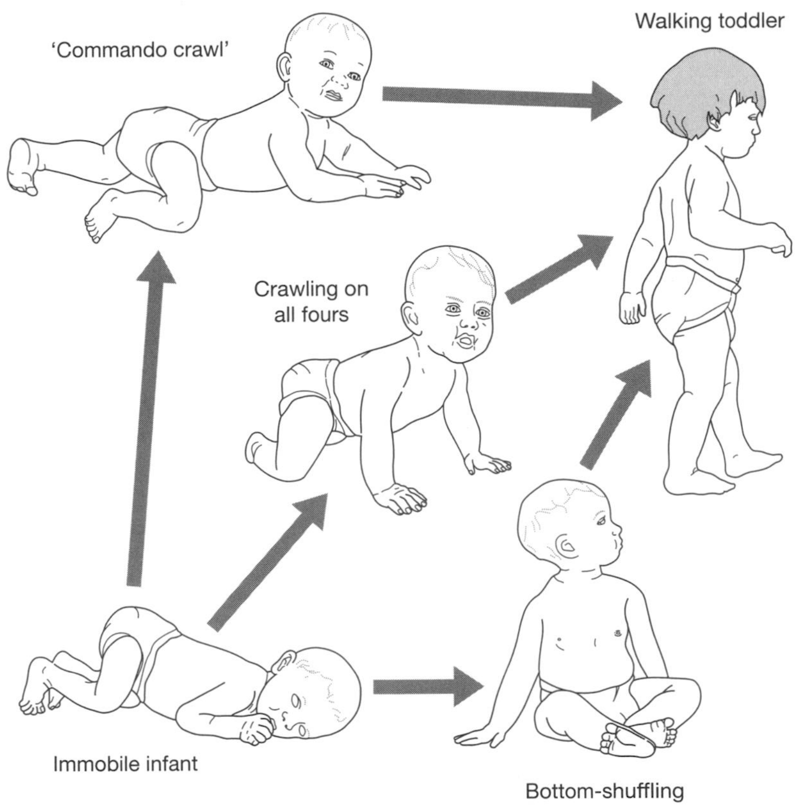

Figure 3.5 The milestones to erect posture

A mature walking pattern is usually achieved by four years of age, and the acquisition of fundamental motor skills progresses rapidly, these being normally attained by 60 per cent of six- to seven-year-olds. Boys tend to attain the skill of throwing and kicking earlier than girls, but girls tend to hop and skip earlier than boys. Fundamental motor skills are climbing, jumping, hopping, skipping, galloping, throwing and catching. It is interesting that children may achieve a mature skill, only to regress while another motor skill is learnt, and then to regain that particular mature skill later (see Chapter 2 for more detail of neuromuscular control).

Development of fine motor skills can be observed as the baby holds a rattle and swipes at nearby objects, whereas the three-year-old can 'colour in' pictures to a greater or lesser extent. The four- to seven-year-old can begin to write its name, thread beads and to play a musical instrument, and the older child increase its sporting abilities as it takes part in team games and activities.

Sleep

Sleep is universal among higher vertebrates and is defined as a state of partial consciousness from which one can be roused by stimulation. This differentiates it from a coma from which one cannot easily be woken. Cortical activity is depressed but brain stem functions such

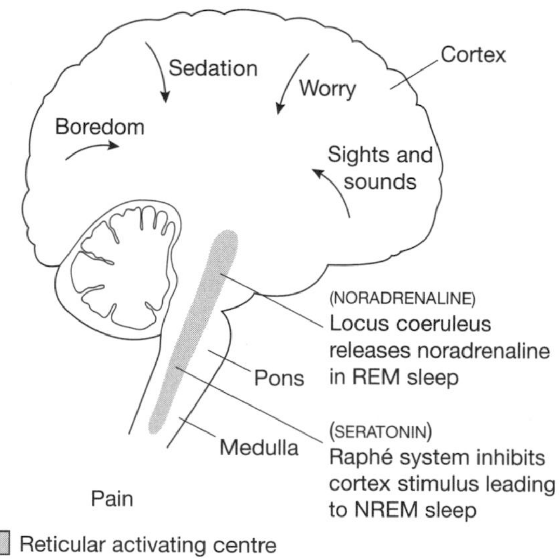

Figure 3.6 The 'sleep centres' of the brain

as control of respiration, heart rate and blood pressure continue (Figure 3.6). Sleep appears vital for survival of brain function. Asleep, children show two very different cyclical phases, and even in the waking state they show these cyclical patterns in high and low activity levels.

Sleep is induced by complex neuro-chemical reactions arising in the tissues of the brain stem known as the reticular formation and mediated by neurotransmitters such as serotonin and noradrenaline. Superimposed on this mechanism are circadian rhythms, which are thought to be controlled by the suprachiasmic nuclei situated near the third ventricle in the brain which connects the retina of the eye to the specialised nerve endings. Our body rhythms are also controlled by external clues, called *zeitgebers*, such as light, dark and daily temperature changes (Bear *et al.* 2007).

Slow wave sleep (SWS or non-REM) is promoted by the Raphé system, and rapid eye movement (REM) sleep is promoted as the activity of neurones in the locus coeruleus increases. The former state is characterised by slow brain waves and movement is observed of body position. In SWS the cerebral metabolic rate is 75 per cent of that when awake; this state is enhanced by the brain being heated during the waking period. Perhaps this is one reason for the child with a fever feeling sleepy or the child who has had a very active day sleeping well at night. Some children are very 'restless' at night in this type of sleep and throw off their covers or fall out of bed, others suffer nightmares where they report frightening situations such as being crushed or suffocated (Carlson 2001). The latter state is quite complex, a paradox, in fact, because the brain appears to be active, cerebral blood flow and oxygen uptake increases and the eyes move under their lids while the body lies very still and skeletal muscles lose their tone. This REM sleep is only observed in warm blooded vertebrates; it is increased in infants and young children as they are learning a lot about their world at a rapid rate, thus they must organise and integrate this with existing memories. Children who are intellectually gifted seem to spend more time in this type of sleep than other children, and retarded children engage in it less. However, those who are deprived of sleep appear to be able to survive adequately, but lack of sleep may have more subtle effects on the child's brain development and learning capacity, especially if it interferes with school performance. Sadeh *et al.* (2002) showed that school-aged children who experienced fragmented sleep did worse on the neuro-function tests for complex activities and had more behaviour problems.

As children mature, the quantity and quality of sleep changes. Family influences, social expectations and cultural variations affect the amount of sleep a child experiences. The total length of time a child sleeps within twenty-four hours decreases throughout childhood; the cycle from SWS to REM sleep increases from forty-five to ninety minutes. Newborn babies sleep for much of the time not occupied with feeding; interestingly, the time intervals are longer the larger the baby is, as the stomach holds more feed and thus satisfies hunger. During the latter part of the first year the baby may sleep all night and also have naps during the day. By the age of two many children will only have a short daytime nap and, by the age of three, most children will not sleep during the day except in cultures where a siesta is customary. From four to ten years the period of night-time sleep shortens slightly but increases again during puberty (Laberge *et al.* 2001).

Sleep can be disrupted by many changes in routine, such as sleeping in a strange bed or being put to bed by an unfamiliar carer. Many researchers have documented these problems and suggested ways to overcome resistance at bedtime. Levin and Neilsen (2007), in their systematic review of disturbed sleep, suggest that sleep problems are common in childhood, and that 50 per cent of children have difficulty settling and experience frequent waking at night. Sadeh (2004) writes that infant sleep problems are the most prevalent problems presented to health care professionals. She suggests that night waking and sleep problems have been associated with difficult temperaments and behaviour problems among children; Levin and Neilson also found correlation with sleep problems and anxiety, with the experience of nightmares related to anxious personality types coping with their personal environmental stressors.

Laberge *et al.* (2001) found that middle adolescents experienced the highest level of sleep disturbance, such as sleep latency, mid-sleep waking and movement during sleep, and suggested that this reflected the changes in hormone activity experienced in puberty. They suggested that reports from girls that they benefited less from their sleep were perhaps due to their earlier hormonal changes and their intuitive reporting of moodiness and level of fatigue. All adolescents showed a higher level of sleep supplementation in the mornings or early evenings; however, the total time in twenty-four hours for all teenagers was consistently in the range 7.8–8 hours. Reasons for these changes in sleep patterns are, perhaps, the expanding social opportunities, academic demands, involvement in part-time jobs and increased access to alcohol and drugs. Investigations into the sleep patterns of the adolescent, such as that of Laberge *et al.* (2001), improve the professional's understanding of some of this age group's special problems and health needs.

Physiology knowledge in practice

Scenario 1

Jimmy, aged twelve months, pulls himself to standing by the armchair in his parent's sitting room. What does his brain have to do for him to achieve this feat?

Some pointers:

- Jimmy has an interest to see new things – he is motivated and his eyes are sending messages via his occipital lobe in the cerebral cortex to his frontal lobe to plan to pull himself up for the investigation. Learning has changed his nervous system circuits in relation to perception, performance, thinking and planning. He is developing useful behaviours that adapt him to his changing environment. Perception uses visual, sound, feel, smell, shape and movement experiences to inform his sensory cortex. He is connecting stimuli and responses as he changes his behaviour to the consequences of his actions – pull on a mobile object and it moves – you do not.
- His memory allows him to recall the fun he had when he tore up the paper yesterday which lay on the seat of this particular chair.
- The motor cortex of his cerebrum activates his skeletal muscles in his legs to contract and move his body up and hold the position by the chair. Feedback from joints, muscles, vestibular apparatus in the ear, information received from the eye and contact with the floor improve the neural circuits in his motor system.
- His cerebellum ensures a detailed sequence of contractions with great precision. Jimmy has practised this for days and is becoming more proficient at remaining upright.
- Jimmy is making relationships between all these stimuli and integrating them into spatial learning and sequential knowledge for future use.

Scenario 2

Ben is ten years old and is moderately affected by cerebral palsy. He has just commenced a course of aromatherapy massage, a complementary therapy, bought for his birthday present by his grandmother. Why do you think this will be beneficial to Ben?

The theory

- Aromatherapy uses essential oils that are readily absorbed through the skin; they are reported to have beneficial effect for muscle spasms, anxiety and other uncomfortable physical symptoms.
- Some essential oils are stimulants and others calming – lavender smell is enjoyed by children but only *lavendula angustifolia* is recommended for this age group. The use of oils must be carefully monitored and best administered with guidance from an experienced practitioner (McNeilly 2004).
- Massage uses the communication of touch – by stimulating the 'slow twitch' fibres it can detract the brain from more painful experiences ('gate theory' of pain physiology). It is a useful distraction skill.
- Massage can encourage the return of lymph fluid from peripheral parts of the body where muscle function is poor. This reduces oedema and improves blood circulation. Ben's poor mobility may result in him suffering swollen feet, especially after long periods of reduced mobility at school.

Extend your knowledge

Read Laberge *et al.*'s 2001 article 'Development of sleep patterns in early adolescents', and talk to your friends and family. Ask them about their sleep activity, such as what time they go to bed and whether this changes at the weekend from school days. See if there is any difference between girls and boys and think about the reasons why the children may have different experiences. Laberge *et al.* did their research with children aged from ten to thirteen years. You might like to extend the age range that you talk to and find out if everyone eventually achieves adult sleep status – whatever that might mean!

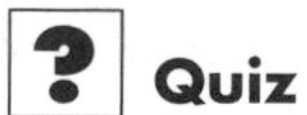

Quiz

1. What is the neural plate?
2. What are the differences between the right and left hemispheres of the brain?
3. What are the primitive general functional areas of the brain?
4. When do the fontanelles of the skull close?
5. When a child is cold how does it generate heat and what would a carer observe in a child who was overheating?
6. Name and give the function of three neuroglial cells.
7. What is the blood/brain barrier?
8. Name some substances that are blocked by the blood/brain barrier.
9. Describe three primitive reflexes you would expect a healthy newborn baby to show.
10. Describe three postural reflexes.
11. Explain why a baby's skin is generally more sensitive than the skin of an older child.
12. Explain why the adolescent needs to start to use deodorants.
13. Why is it important that a child's strabismus (squint) is corrected before the age of four years?
14. Describe the mechanism for hearing sound.
15. What are the 'language' sounds you would expect to hear from a child of four to seven months?
16. What does cephalocaudal development mean?
17. What affects a child's motor development?
18. How is sleep different to coma?
19. How is the sleep circadian rhythm controlled?
20. What are the chemicals of sleep?

Further reading

Tanner, J.M. (1989) *Foetus into Man: Physical Growth from Conception to Maturity* (2nd edition), Ware: Castlemead.

Chapter 4

The cardiovascular system

- Heart embryology
- Foetal heart circulation
- Blood cell production in the foetus and neonate
- Children's blood
- Common blood tests
- Circulation changes in the heart at birth
- Changes in the cardiovascular system in childhood
- Exercise and cardiovascular function

THE NORMAL RESTING metabolism needs adequate body perfusion of blood to service the rising energy requirements in children as they grow. This must be matched by similar improvements in cardiac output. Basic metabolic rate (BMR), related to the increasing body mass and relative decrease of surface area, becomes increasingly inversely related to body size. Resting BMR must be matched to cardiac output for healthy growth. The heart develops from two tubes lying side by side and it is the complex changes in this muscle pump as it develops that gives rise to the eventual double circulation in the heart: receiving blood from the body systems and re-oxygenating it in the lungs before delivering it back to the body tissues (see Figure 4.1).

Heart embryology

A common problem, soon after birth, is cardiac abnormality. An overview of the development of the heart will advise on the usual signs and symptoms of malfunction.

In the fourth week after conception a pair of angioblastic cords develop from the mesoderm to form a pair of endocardial tubes,

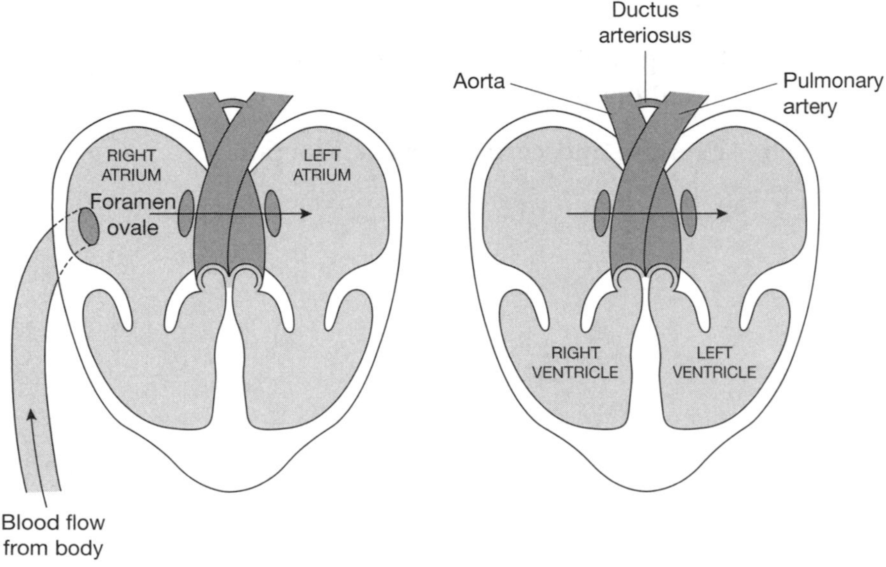

Figure 4.1 Foramen ovale and ductus arteriosis

which then fuse to form the primitive heart tube. This starts to beat on day twenty-two, shunting blood round the embryo by day twenty-four. Between weeks five and eight this tube remodels to transform into four chambers. In the fifth week septi grow to separate the right and left atria, and the valves between the atria and septi form. The right atrial fibre tract develops to form the heart pacemaker, as up to this time the heart has 'beaten' due to myogenic stimulus as the blood flowed through tubes whose walls contain myocytes enervated by the autonomic nervous system. The ventricles are separated by the eighth week; this last intricate remoulding is vital, with most common defects at birth being found here.

Starting from day seventeen, spaces occur in the splanchnic mesoderm and blood vessels begin to arise from the yolk sac wall 'blood islands' that interconnect and develop into the endothelium of the primitive blood and lymph circulation. Valves in veins are present at six months of foetal life. Lymphatic channels arise in the fifth embryonic week (Moore 2003). Primitive blood cells arise within the yolk sac and the extra-embryonic mesoderm associated with the chorion (Marieb and Hoehn 2007). Blood cell production on day eighteen switches from the yolk sac to the liver, spleen, thymus and finally the bone marrow.

Foetal heart circulation

Oxygenation for the foetus occurs in the placenta, an inefficient oxygenation system, that bypasses the foetal lungs by using a short cut passage through the heart. The foetus is always hypoxic with an aortic arterial oxygenation saturation of 60 to 70 per cent. To maintain adequate oxygen delivery, foetal cardiac output is thus higher, at 440–500 ml/kg/min, than in the neonate in order to maintain blood supply to the foetal brain. In the foetal circulation oxygenated blood enters the body through the left umbilical vein. It then mixes with a small volume of deoxygenated blood that is returning from the portal system, legs and lower body trunk in the inferior vena cava. The flow moves up to the right atrium, where the pressure is higher than the left ventricle as it receives all the blood from the systemic return and placenta. It then flows to the left atrium through the foramen ovale in a distinct stream alongside the deoxygenated blood from the superior vena cava, draining blood from the head and upper trunk (Figure 4.2). Here, there is a little mixing with the small amount of blood that has circulated to nourish the developing pulmonary tissue, before it returns to the placenta via the pulmonary veins. Pulmonary resistance is very high in the foetal lung fields as they are filled with fluid. This fluid, rather than air filling, results in the hypoxic alveoli stimulating pulmonary vessel vasoconstriction. Most of the returning superior vena cava blood moves into the right ventricle, which would then normally flow round the lungs in the pulmonary circulation. In the foetus only some of this blood moves up the pulmonary artery towards the lungs; the rest is diverted into the ductus arteriosus which bypasses the lungs to the descending aorta. The still well-oxygenated blood is then propelled to the foetus's body tissues via the aorta which offer little vascular resistance, before returning to the placenta via the umbilical artery for oxygenation.

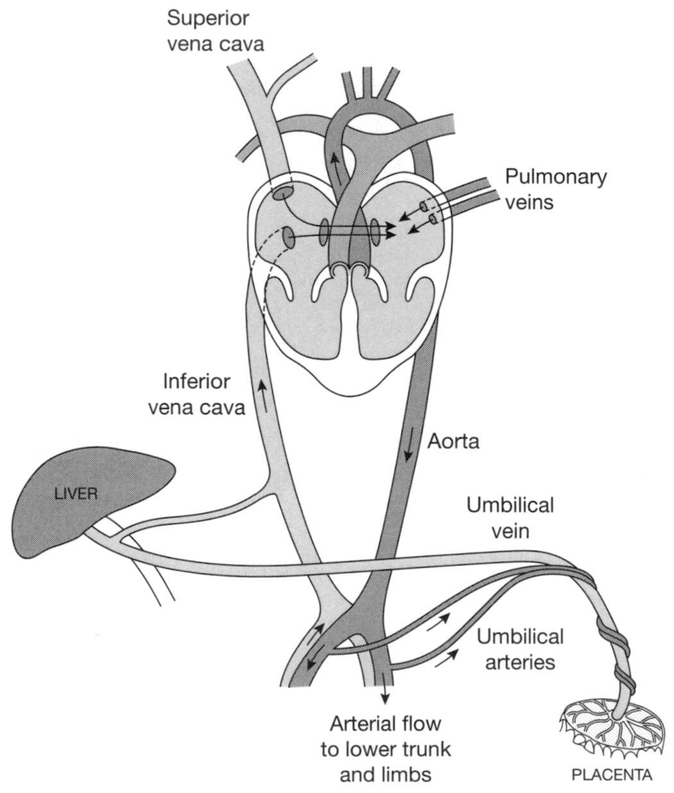

Figure 4.2 Foetal circulation

Blood cell production in the foetus and neonate

The foetus has a boost to its oxygen carrying capacity in that its red blood cells are formed differently for its time in the uterus. One of the factors that favours oxygen diffusion across the placenta to the developing foetus is that the haemoglobin type HbF, produced in utero, is not affected by the 2.3DPG present in the adult red cells to induce offloading to tissues. Therefore, the foetal haemoglobin oxygen curve shows slightly greater oxygen affinity than does that of the mother. Also the haemoglobin concentration in the foetal blood is high, 15–23 g/dl 200 g/l, so the foetus's arterial blood has nearly the same oxygen concentration as that of its mother, even though its arterial oxygen pressure is less than 40 mm mercury. At birth this still remains high at 18 g/dl.

Foetal blood cells are formed on the surface of the yolk sac fourteen to nineteen days after conception; this process then continues until the third trimester of the pregnancy. At the same time haemopoiesis commences in the liver, spleen and bone marrow, the latter being the major producer at twenty-six weeks. After twenty-eight weeks a switch to HbA occurs and at birth, the ratio of HbF to HbA is 80:20. At six months of age there is normally only 1 per cent of HbF present (Baker 2006) as it has been rapidly destroyed by the liver. However, on the first day of life the HbF levels rise due to extracellular fluid loss during labour and birth; it then reduces until two to three months of age to the normal lower limit (9.5 g/dl). This initial slow rate of red blood cell production occurs because of an immaturity of neonate bone marrow which develops capacity over the first six months of extra-uterine life.

Later anaemia in children is usually related to dietary iron deficiency, and is diagnosed by observation of pallor and pica (eating non-food materials such as paper). The current recommendation in the UK is to commence weaning at six months and to supplement the feeds with iron before this time if the infant is bottle-fed on cow's milk. Breastfed babies can extract 50 per cent of their iron needs whereas bottle-fed babies can only extract 10 per cent from cow's milk. Thus, a substitute milk feed formula has iron added. By the age of one year the fast growing child will require good supplies of iron rich foods; they need 8 mg/day – half of that required by their mother.

Children's blood

The average blood volume in the full-term infant is 85 ml/kg. Red cells are made in the red bone marrow which occupies most of the spongy spaces and long bone cavities of the skeleton in childhood. However, by puberty red marrow is partially replaced by yellow containing fat, and red cell production only remains in the upper shaft of the femur and humerus, vertebrae, sternum, ribs, innominate bones and scapulae. The bone marrow is particularly active when there has been blood loss; it increases activity to boost the red cell count. For red cell production the red marrow must have supplies of amino acids, iron, vitamins B12 and B6, and folic acid. Thus, the child's diet is crucial to healthy blood formation (Table 4.1). Red marrow is stimulated to become active by erythopoietin, a hormone secreted from the kidney, and also by thyroxine, androgens and growth hormone. In emergencies the marrow can show a tenfold increase in productivity. In the three-month foetus, reticulocytes are 90 per cent of the red cell blood count but drop to 2–7 per cent in the newborn and 0.5–1.5 per cent at three days of extra-uterine life. Reticulocytes are immature red cells that circulate in the blood and mature in two days. In the adult they make up 0.8 per cent of the blood cells.

Table 4.1 Normal haematology in childhood

Age	*Hb (g/dl)*	*MCV (fl)*	*WBC (10^9/l)*	*Plats*
Birth	14.5–21.5	100–135	10.0–26.0	150–450
2 weeks	13.4–19.8	88–120	6.0–21.0	150–450
2 months	9.4–13.0	84–105	6.0–18.0	150–450
1 year	11.3–14.1	71–85	6.0–17.5	150–450
2–6 years	11.5–13.5	75–87	5.0–17.0	150–450
6–12 years	11.5–15.5	77–95	4.5–14.5	150–450
Male adult	13.0–16.0	78–95	4.5–13.0	150–450
Female adult	12.0–16.0	78–95	4.5–13.0	150–450

Source: Lissauer and Clayden 2004.

Note: Hb g/dl = haemoglobin (grams per decilitre). MCV = mean red cell volume. WBC = white blood cell. Plats = blood platelets.

Common blood tests

Babies are tested soon after birth for common genetic conditions by blood tests, the symptoms of which can be improved with prior knowledge.

Guthrie test

This is to test for high levels of phenylalanine found in 1:7,000–10,000 live births. It is a genetic autosomal recessive disorder. Excess of this chemical in the blood shows that the child's liver is not converting phenyalanine to tyrosine, an essential amino acid for tissue growth. Phenylketanuria (PKU) will lead to brain damage if undetected and not treated with an adjusted protein diet from birth. The child will usually be tested by heel prick on the sixth day of life after milk feeds have been established (www.nspku.org).

At the same time as the Guthrie test, the child will be tested from the same heel prick sample for hypothyroidism, which is seen in 1:4,000 infants. This is a congenital condition where, if not treated with replacement hormone which is essential for the development of brain and bones, cretinism develops (www.screening.nhs.uk, www.newbornscreening.bloodspot.org.uk).

Routine vitamin supplement after birth

Some recommendations for food supplements are made universally for all children in the UK. This is in response to known preventable disabling conditions. Other extra recommendations will then be made in relation to individual need such as multivitamins for the premature infant or sodium supplements in some congenital metabolic diseases.

Vitamin K

The newborn has two mechanisms for preventing bleeding. These are platelets and coagulation factors:

- At birth, platelets are 150–450 × 10^9/l and remain stable for life (Thureen *et al.* 2004).

- Coagulation factors are synthesised in the liver and depend on adequate vitamin K levels. These are low at birth and drop further in the first few days of life. Vitamin K is normally made in the gut by bacteria, but at birth the gut is sterile and only gradually becomes colonised during feeding, taking longer in breastfed babies than those who are bottle-fed.

Vitamin K supplement is considered important to guard against intracranial bleeding after delivery; 0.5 mg is given orally (or 0.1 mg intramuscularly/intravenously) to all babies within the first hour of birth to promote hepatic biosynthesis of vitamin K. Two more doses of 0.5 mg are given at seven days and six weeks. The intramuscular route is preferred as this vitamin is poorly absorbed from the gut.

Circulation changes in the heart at birth

At birth the heart occupies 40 per cent of the lung fields (30 per cent in adults). Changes in the foetal circulation at birth occur as babies start to depend on their lungs for oxygen rather than blood flow from their mother's placenta.

The Apgar score, taken at one minute and five minutes after birth, is scored for a pulse which is either absent (zero points), or lower than 100 (one point) or above 100 (two points). The score is added to scores from other critical measurements (linked to respiratory, muscular skeletal and nervous systems) and together they predict satisfactory survival of the infant. However, the baby may look blue at the extremities for a few hours after birth until peripheral circulation is established (Table 4.2).

Table 4.2 Apgar score sheet

Score	*0*	*1*	*2*
Heart rate	Absent	<100 beats/min	>100 beats/min
Respiratory effort	Absent	Gasping/irregular	Regular/strong cry
Muscle tone	Flaccid	Some flexion of limbs	Well flexed/active
Reflex irritability	None	Grimace	Cry/cough
Colour	Pale/blue	Body pink/extremities blue	Pink

Source: Lissauer and Clayden 2004.

At birth, when the infant takes its first breath, the alveoli in the lungs fill with air and the constricted pulmonary vessels open to allow more blood to flow to the lungs. At the same time umbilical flow is halted. The heart rate is approximately 140 beats per minute in the first fifteen minutes and then reduces to a 90–175 range depending on external stimuli and activity level. The pressure changes, and reduction of prostaglandin E and prostacyclin (which act as local vasodilators) which maintain the pregnancy, cause the *ductus arteriosis* and *foramen ovale* to close. This happens over the first ten to fifteen hours of extra-uterine life in the full term baby. The newborn may exhibit a soft systolic murmur which will disappear as the cardiac circulation adapts to pressure changes in circulation. Hepatic flow, ensured by the umbilical vein and also kept patent by prostaglandins in the foetus, is taken over by the portal system within a few days after birth (Figure 4.3). Oxygen consumption doubles from 7–8 ml/kg/min to 15–18 ml/kg/min at this time; thus, a corresponding ventricular output is seen. Oxygen demand remains high, and anything that increases oxygen demand, for example cold or sepsis, will stress the baby's heart. At eight weeks post-natal oxygen consumption drops by 50 per cent.

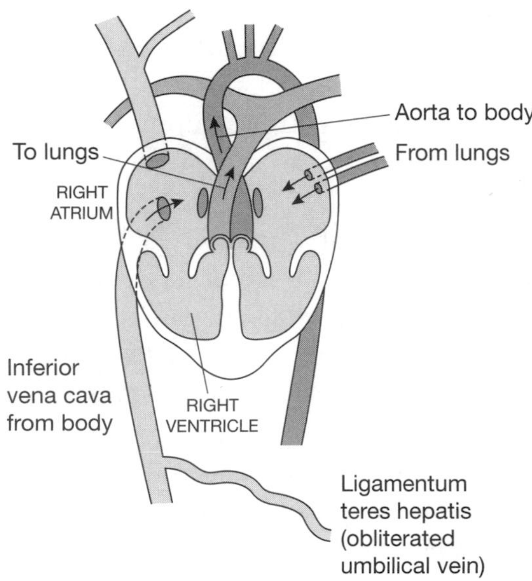

Figure 4.3 Circulation after birth

Changes in the cardiovascular system in childhood

The mass of the heart as a ratio of the total body mass is high in babies but reduces as childhood progresses. The newborn heart has right ventricle dominance with right thickening in the muscle wall but, as pulmonary resistance falls in change from foetal circulation, it thins. At four weeks the right ventricle equals the left ventricle in weight. The heart weight doubles in the first year of life and has grown six-fold by the age of nine (McCance and Heuther 2006). There is a 20 per cent decline in growth rate from three to fifteen years. The left ventricle mass closely relates to body surface area. La Place's law requires that a rise in blood pressure with age is matched by a proportionately greater ratio of wall thickness to chamber dimensions to maintain constant wall stress. Over childhood cardiac muscle fibres increase seven times in size, with cardiac blood vessels increasing in number to supply them; however, small babies have greater myocardial contractility than older children. Cardiac ability rises with age, but children's and adolescents' cardiac outputs are lower than those of adults at any given level of oxygen uptake. Cardiac output is related to heart rate and stroke volume (Table 4.3). Children's smaller hearts (stroke volume) beat faster (rate) to oxygenate their body tissues. Resting stroke volume is related to body weight, but this is influenced by body composition, for example, lean body mass. Children of different sizes have different normal ranges of cardiac output, thus the cardiac index (CI) is often used for them:

> CI = CO divided by body surface in metres squared (normal is 3.5–4.5 $l/min/m^2$ of body surface)

Any increase in normal rate, however, does not improve overall cardiac function. With over 200–220 beats per minute in infants and 160–180 beats per minute in children, one would see a ventricular diastolic filling time and coronary artery perfusion time reduced, leading to a fall in stroke volume and cardiac output. In fact, transient bradicardia may then occur which leads to a fall in systemic perfusion; the child becomes mottled and pale in colour; peripheral vasoconstriction occurs; peripheral extremities become cool; there is delayed capillary refill; decreased urine output is seen; and a metabolic acidosis is evident. Interestingly, arterial systolic blood pressure may remain normal as the result of arterial constriction.

Table 4.3 Normal paediatric cardiac output (CO): stroke volume (SV)

Age	*Pulse*	*CO l/min*	*SV*
Newborn	145	0.8–1.0	5
6 months	120	1.0–1.3	10
1 year	115	1.3–1.5	13
5 years	95	2.5–3.0	31
10 years	75	3.8–4.0	50
15 years	70	6.0	85

Source: Halazinski 1992.

A fat child's cardiac output may, therefore, be underestimated. However, obesity in children cannot be well defined, due to their total body water and reduced bone density. Body fat to skin fat ratio is higher anyway in children. Heart rate falls in childhood (Table 4.4); from nine years gender effects are also seen. (Basal rates are those measured twelve hours after a meal and with the subject having rested for thirty minutes.) Food consumption, anxiety and anticipatory neurohormonal changes, such as fright, also change heart rate. Thus, basal measurements for children are difficult to calculate when they are awake.

Heart rate measurements over childhood reflect a decreasing basic metabolic rate (BMR is related to mass and surface area – the smaller the child the greater the BMR as they have a relatively large surface area to body mass). In females this drops 23 per cent from the ages of six to sixteen years; their resting heart rate also reduces over this time by 20 per cent. The growing child shows a decreasing BMR and a rise in heart stroke volume. As their heart grows in size and the nerve networks to the cardiac muscle mature, the volume of blood they can expel per heart beat increases; where physical activity is regularly encouraged the heart should grow in size to its healthy maximum.

Wallis *et al.* (2005) offer discussion on methods for taking a pulse rate as having a stimulating effect on children and suggest that published ranges of normal pulse rates should be used with caution and the child's situation at the time of the measurement given due consideration. For example, if one applies a finger probe to take a pulse rate the child may fear the monitor and their

Table 4.4 Heart rates in childhood

Age	*Rate*
Under 1 year	110–160
2–5 years	95–140
5–12 years	80–120
Over 12 years	60–100

Source: Lissauer and Clayden 2004.

physiological response may cloud the true reading. Interestingly, Wallis and Maconochie (2006) found little difference in pulse range in healthy South African children aged five to sixteen years who suffered social deprivation; the family circumstances of the children had no obvious effect on their developing cardiovascular system.

Exercise and cardiovascular function

Pulse rate will rise as exercise increases because the heart volume (size) will remain the same but the blood will need to move faster to take oxygen to the active cells in the muscles. The younger the child, the smaller the heart so they show a higher pulse rate at any given level of activity. Pulse rates rise on physical effort and in other situations where metabolic rate is increased, such as fever and anxiety. Children's maximal heart rates are higher than adults; they may rise to a rate of approximately 200 beats per minute depending on their age and size. All girls have similar maximal heart rates at the same age but significantly higher rates sub-maximally than similar aged boys. These differences appear at about the age of six years.

Children's response to exercise is related to their age, the type of exercise undertaken and the gradual effect of physical activity in their day to day life. Armstrong (2006) gives comprehensive information on young people who have a more favourable peripheral distribution of blood during exercise, facilitating the transport of oxygen to the exercising muscles. Children have a slightly higher mitochondrial density and oxidative enzyme availability than adults, and thus have an increased ability to change sugar to energy in the working muscle cell. The cardiac output of children may be much lower at the same oxygen uptake compared to adults but the child relies on higher peripheral oxygen extraction ability in the muscles themselves. At gentle exercise levels, increased oxygen extraction from the blood can compensate for the low cardiac output. At more strenuous levels this advantage is limited by their lower haemoglobin content of the blood to transport oxygen to the tissues. They recover from exercise more quickly than adults because their smaller muscle effort is lower at any given activity.

Although there are no differences in early childhood, boys show an increasing haemoglobin concentration as they grow older when testosterone has an increasing effect on the growth spurt and development of secondary sexual characteristics such as greater muscle mass in their late teens. Girls, on the other hand, show a lower increase in haemoglobin levels by menarche; thus teenage boys show superiority in endurance events because their blood is able to carry oxygen more efficiently to bigger working muscles.

Resting blood pressure rises throughout childhood as the heart becomes bigger and stronger (see Table 4.5). Children of eight to ten years of age also demonstrate an ultradian rhythm, and that the development and maturity of the cardiovascular system and the underlying neurological mechanisms may be a prerequisite to the achievement of adult blood pressure circadian rhythm, which would show a twenty-four-hour period (Marieb and Hoehn 2007). Measurement of a child's blood pressure can be an inexact science as they become anxious when their arm or leg is compressed, the correct cuff bladder is also vital as systolic readings can be raised as much as 20 mmHg and hypertension erroneously diagnosed (Summers 2007).

Table 4.5 Blood pressure changes over childhood

Age	*Male*	*Female*
1 year	80/34–89/39	83/38–90/42
5 years	90/50–98/55	89/52–96/56
10 years	97/58–106/63	98/59–105/62
15 years	109/61–117/66	107/64–113/67

Note: Reference adapted from American Academy of Pediatrics website, www.aap.org/topics.html. Values given reflect the fifth to ninety-fifth centile range of height in mm-Hg at rest.

Peripheral resistance factors such as sympathetic enervation of blood vessels, blood viscosity changes and local muscle response to metabolites are poorly researched at present. However, arterial blood vessels in children under one year have been found to contain fatty streaks regardless of sex, race, geography or hereditary factors, and these appear in the coronary arteries of children aged ten years. Studies have shown that 26 per cent of children in the two- to twelve-year age group have raised serum cholesterol (above the 5.2 mmol/l recognised as the maximum desirable). By the early teens, Jackson *et al.* (2006) found pulse pressure peaking before a drop as they enter young adult life – a phenomenon they could not explain. The pulse pressure is the difference between systolic and diastolic pressure readings; a greater difference is indicative of cardiovascular morbidity such as hypertension and atheroma. Hippisley-Cox *et al.* (2007) offer risk predictions for cardiovascular disease (CVD) that include social deprivation, family history of CVD, raised BMI (ratio of height to weight – see Table 4.4 where blood pressure (B/P) range is related to height), high blood pressure outside the accepted range and smoking. Whether atheroma lesions are reversible or precursors of more permanent fibrous plaques may be influenced by subsequent 'risky' behaviour as offered by Hippisley-Cox *et al.*; they may have an early effect in childhood on peripheral resistance and thus a long-term risk factor of a rising blood pressure. Weight control, regular exercise and a diet low in animal fats have been shown to reduce serum cholesterol in all age groups and reduce the risk of CVD in the population.

Physiology knowledge in practice

Scenario 1

Maisie is three days old and is the first child of Jack and Diana who are both aged seventeen. Maisie appears well but has slight yellowing of her sclera. They are worried that the vitamin K injection Maisie had after she was born caused her to become jaundiced. What can you tell them and what advice could you give?

Some pointers:

- Vitamin K will prevent Maisie from suffering an intracranial bleed as she has only 30 to 60 per cent of this vitamin and other clotting factors stored in her body at birth. Fat soluble vitamin K is used by the liver to synthesise coagulation factors 11, V11, 1X and X. Spontaneous haemorrhage from the umbilical cord and intestinal mucosa occurs in babies when the stored vitamin K obtained from the mother before birth has been used up and the intestinal bacteria needed for its synthesis in the baby's bowel are not yet established. Adult levels of clotting factors are achieved by six weeks of post-natal life. Maisie has none of the symptoms of vitamin K deficiency.

- Jaundice is common in the newborn. The liver enzymes function at 60 per cent of normal activity level at three days old; red cells containing HbF are being broken down rapidly and bile, which is the waste product of their destruction, is re-absorbed from the gut because of the low gut flora, slow gut motility and small enteral (milk) intake. Maisie's colour should improve as she increases her feeds.
- Her mother should be encouraged to feed her on demand and observe for green stools which will show the bile being excreted from her body. As the bile levels reduce her stool colour will change to yellow.
- The parents should also watch Maisie for feeding and sleeping activity; if she appears drowsy or not hungry they should ask for professional help.

Scenario 2

Peter, aged twelve, has recently been fainting in assembly at school. What knowledge would help his teachers to an understanding of this problem?

The theory

- Syncope (fainting) is caused by: neurocardiogenic instability – disturbance of heart rate and blood pressure controls; cardiovascular abnormalities; epilepsy and psychogenic causes.
- McLeod (2003) reports that the first reason for syncope is very common in childhood. It usually occurs when the child is upright – sitting or standing. Peter may have been asked to stand for lengthy periods in a crowded hall. The child shows dizziness, nausea and pallor before loss of tone and consciousness. As the

brain is starved of oxygen from hypotenstion (low B/P) or bradycardia (slow heart beat) it may have had an anoxic seizure (the child becomes stiff and may twitch) and may become incontinent.

- Baroreceptors in the blood circulation system control arteriole size – they respond to low blood pressure by constricting and redirecting blood flow to the brain and heart from the periphery of the body. Thus Peter will look pale. If the blood volume is too low the flow will not be adequate to perfuse the vital organs such as the brain and heart. Peter will feel dizzy and his pulse rate will rise and he will eventually lose consciousness. He will fall to the horizontal position where blood flow can then reach his brain and his pulse rate will fall as his heart will not have to pump blood to his head against gravity.
- If Peter has a slow heart beat, inadequate blood volume of oxygenated blood will be pumped to the brain so he will, again, feel dizzy and look pale. The brain will malfunction – he will lose consciousness, electrical activity will become random as he may suffer a seizure, and control of his bladder and bowel will be lost until he recovers.
- Cardiac output depends on both the heart pumping enough blood to the circulation (heart rate) and the resistance of the blood vessels carrying that blood to perfuse the body organs.
- The main treatment is reassurance that the child is not epileptic or has severe cardiac abnormalities. (In repeated fainting episodes the child may be referred for an ECG – electrocardiogram – to check no heart abnormalities are present and/or an EEG – electroencephalogram – to check for brain abnormalities.) Advice should be given to drink plenty of fluids to increase blood volume and increase dietary salt which will raise the blood pressure by retaining the fluid in the circulatory system.
- Some children may faint due to pain, such as those female teenagers suffering a difficult menarche, others may faint due to overriding emotions such as shock or lack of glucose (breakfast!) for brain function. All cells of the body need oxygen and glucose to make energy for activity – the brain is most sensitive to inadequate supplies.
- When fainting feelings are felt, crossing legs and folding arms will help maintain blood pressure. This tenses the muscles in the periphery of the body and presses on the veins to increase the blood flow back to the heart and thus increase blood volume for

pumping to the core organs. Active tension and other bio-feedback techniques such as tilt training are helpful (see McLeod's 2003 paper for details).

Extend your knowledge

Researchers Boreham *et al.* (2001) examined 1,015 schoolchildren between the ages of twelve and fifteen and measured their height, weight, pubertal status, skin fold thickness, blood pressure, blood and fitness status under standardised conditions, when researching their article 'Fitness, fatness and coronary heart disease risk in adolescents'. What was their argument for weight control to prevent cardiovascular disease and what do you consider the causes to be for weight gain in the UK adolescent group?

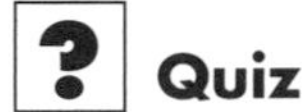

Quiz

1 When does the heart start to develop after conception?
2 From which blood vessel does the foetus receive oxygenated blood?
3 Which vessel takes blood to the placenta for re-oxygenation?
4 What is the haemoglobin level of the neonate?
5 What is the current recommendation in the UK on iron intake for babies and is there different advice for bottle and breastfed babies?
6 What is the average blood volume of a newborn baby?
7 What must a child's diet include for red cell production?
8 What is the Guthrie test?
9 What is the platelet count at birth?
10 What is the Apgar score for the CVS and what other critical measurements must be taken?
11 What is the cardiac index?
12 What would you observe if the child has reduced cardiac perfusion?

13 Why do children's pulse rates decrease as they get older?

14 What is the normal range of pulse rate for a two- to five-year-old child?

15 What effects a child's physical response to exercise?

16 Why do teenage boys do better at endurance activities than teenage girls?

17 What is the average B/P range for a ten-year-old boy?

18 Why is measurement of B/P an inexact science on children?

19 What are CVD risk factors for children?

20 How can parents reduce the risk of CVD in their children?

Chapter 5

The respiratory system

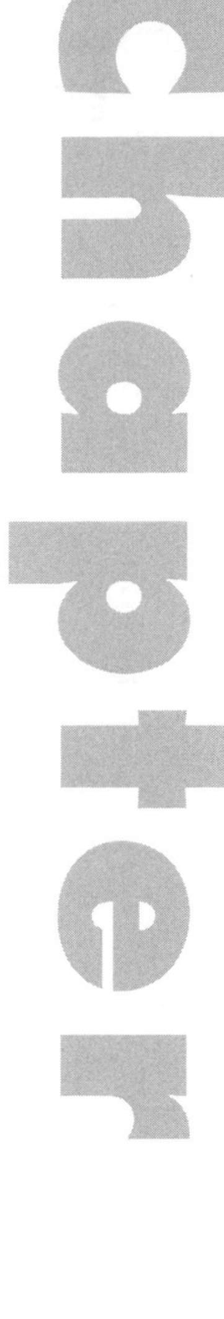

- Embryology
- Surfactant
- The lungs at birth
- Infant breathing – the first few weeks
- The small child's breathing
- Apnoea
- Respiratory resuscitation
- Changes at puberty
- Measuring respiratory rates
- Respiration during exercise
- Breathing changes during sleep
- Development of the ear

HEALTHY SPONTANEOUS BREATHING is normally quiet and accomplished without effort. The amount of energy expended on breathing depends on the rate and depth of each breath, airway resistance and compliance (stretch) of the lungs. An easy revision aid can be found at www.blobs.org/science/anatomy. Figure 5.1 shows the normal respiratory system anatomy. The ribs, intercostal muscles and diaphragm allow ventilation (the moving of air in and out of the lungs) under the control of the respiratory centre in the brain and the lung sacs (the alveoli) allow oxygen and carbon dioxide gases to exchange with the blood.

In the term infant there is a transition of breathing from episodic irregular, ineffectual movements to regular, rhythmic and effectual effort which is completed by the end of the first week of life. Respiratory rate, at seven days of age, will then show a response, increasing as does the adult response, to hypoxaemia (low oxygen levels in the blood). Thus the main adaptation from maternal blood supply to

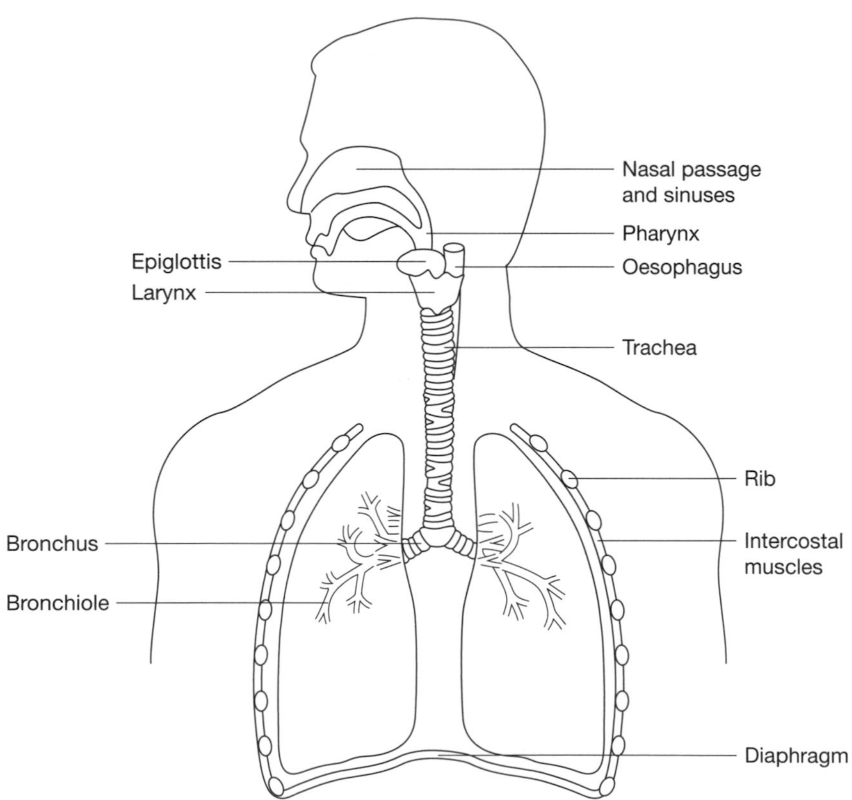

Figure 5.1 Respiratory system

air breathing has occurred by the end of week one. The respiratory system then grows and matures until eight years of age when the 'respiratory tree' is completed. After this age environmental effects and changes in other body systems, especially those affected by sex hormones during puberty, may affect an individual child's eventual adult respiratory function.

Embryology

Lung structure growth and development continues through the foetal and post-natal period, the embryonic stage commencing in the fourth gestational week on day twenty-two when lungs appear as a bud from the oesophagus below the pharyngeal pouches at week five (Marieb and Hoehn 2007). Two branches, the bronchi, bud out on day twenty-six to twenty-eight, the right being larger than the left and orientated more vertically (Figure 5.2).

By the eighth week more branching has occurred from the bronchi, and hyaline cartilage is evident in their walls together with smooth muscle and capillaries. At seventeen weeks' gestation all structures are formed; the lung endoderm branching has occurred sixteen times to produce terminal bronchioles, but no gas exchange is possible, thus the foetus would not be viable if delivered at this stage. From sixteen to twenty-five weeks terminal bronchioles become highly vascular, terminal sacs become thin-walled and some gas exchange is possible. Infants in this age range can survive, but they differ in their individual ability to do so. Under twenty-four weeks' gestation, they have such immature lungs that they are at risk of permanent lung damage. In 2007, however, some survived with adequately

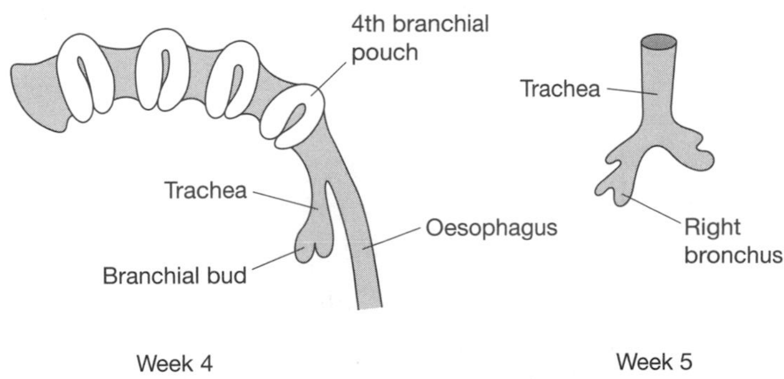

Figure 5.2 Lung buds at week four and bronchi at week five

functioning lungs due to advances in neonatal medicine interventions. From twenty-four weeks to birth the terminal sacs develop and the pulmonary circulation continues to align to the terminal air saccules and increase the area for gas exchange (Aylott 2006). About twenty to seventy million alveoli are formed in each lung by birth; the total number in the adult will reach 300–400 million.

Foetal pulmonary resistance is very high; the lungs are filled with fluid so the alveoli are hypoxic and no gas exchange can take place (the mechanism for blood vessels round the lung to open and close is related to the availability of oxygen in the alveoli). This ensures that pulmonary vasoconstriction remains and only 8 per cent of the total blood volume flows into the lung field – enough to nourish the developing pulmonary tissue only (see Chapter 4 on the cardiovascular system). This hypoxia also leads to reduced breathing movements (ventilation); the reduction in muscle movement reduces the overall oxygen demand of the foetus. Normally ventilation rate responds to the amount of oxygen and carbon dioxide in the blood that passes through the 'breathing control centre in the brain' – the medulla and pons. In the uterus, the foetus's blood is oxygenated via the placenta from the mother so the foetus's 'breathing control centre' interprets its blood as adequately oxygenated and increased breathing movements are not initiated. At twenty weeks' gestation, the bronchi and bronchioles' musculature is complete. After this, muscle increases in the pulmonary arteries and the capillary beds and completes their development round the terminal acinae of the alveoli. This increasing elasticity leads to a reduction of pulmonary resistance in the third trimester of pregnancy ready for birth and the use of oxygen gas for blood exchange. The foetus shows frequent, shallow, irregular breathing movements from the second half of the pregnancy; its thoracic musculature will move in REM sleep for half to one-third of the time (Baker 2006).

Surfactant

Surfactant is vital to keep the small air sacs open in the lungs; without this secretion the lungs collapse, become scarred and have a smaller capacity to move oxygen to the blood. It is secreted from the type two pneumocytes in the alveoli walls. This counteracts surface tension forces and facilitates further terminal sac development.

Surfactant is a detergent-like complex of lipids and proteins that is secreted on to the alveoli surface. This prevents the sacs from collapsing on expiration because it reduces surface tension on their internal surface; it maintains the functional residual capacity (Aylott 2006). Water is the major component of the liquid film that covers the alveoli walls. Where water contacts gases, its molecules bind tightly together and produce a tension that collapses the air sacs. Surfactant mixes with the water and loosens the cohesive tension at the film surface which reduces the pull to collapse the sacs and makes it easier for them to expand with air.

At twenty-two weeks' gestation surfactant is being secreted, with a surge in its production at thirty to thirty-five weeks and at birth. It flows up the trachea out of the mouth into the amniotic fluid; it can be tested by amniocentesis of the mother. Its production is reduced by intrapartum asphyxia from antepartum haemorrhage or maternal hypotension. Increase is promoted when the maternal membranes have ruptured for more than twenty-four hours in preparation for birth, placental infarction has occurred in pre-eclampsia, or when hypertension with intrauterine growth retardation is evident. Stress to the foetus in these situations causes gluco-corticoids to be released from the adrenal glands, and these also stimulate surfactant release to prepare the infant for extra-uterine life (Baker 2006). Today, mothers in premature labour may be treated with betamethasone (a steroid) to protect their infants' lungs and small, premature babies may be given surfactant through their ventilator endotracheal tube with good effect.

The lungs at birth

The lungs of the foetus are filled with fluid until delivery. As the baby is squeezed through the vaginal canal the lungs are gradually squeezed free of fluid, but the baby may need suction to remove residual mucus from the mouth and nose before it is swallowed. Residual fluid is absorbed through the pulmonary capillaries and into the lymphatic vessels which return it to the inferior vena cava veins and thus to the heart. Mild cooling, light, sound, touch, odours and added gravity force, combined with the internal stimuli of reduced blood oxygen and rising carbon dioxide levels in the blood (increasing acidity), stimulate the respiratory centre in the brain and the infant should then take its first breath of air. Once the lungs are taking in air they will not refill with fluid. As the lungs expand, mechanical effects on the pulmonary arterioles, and changes in the blood flow pressures in the heart, allow them to dilate and blood flows to the capillary networks round the alveoli in the lungs. The lungs recoil away from the chest wall due to the elastic fibres in the lung tissue, and the chest wall springs out. Healthy lung compliance (ability to stretch) then is determined by the amount of surfactant reducing alveoli surface tension and elasticity of the alveoli.

Infant breathing – the first few weeks

The infant has low oxygen levels in the blood at birth, and its breathing shows a transitory biphasic structure; at first, ventilation responds to low oxygen but then drops to prehypoxic levels or below. This phenomenon adjusts to an adult response by day seven. The delayed response may be due to immature mechanical factors involving the lungs and chest wall, immature respiratory-related neurotransmitter systems in the brain and an immature peripheral arterial chemosensor system. In the first days of life the neonate also demonstrates intrapulmonary shunting of blood due to the alveoli having some blocked and oedematous areas remaining. The poor perfusion of these sections of lung tissue results in a certain amount of hypoxaemia. Thus the oxygen pressures in the blood at day one may be 80 mmHg and not peak to 95+ mmHg for seven days. However, the carbon dioxide and blood acidity appear within normal range over this time. In the pre-term birth, however, an infant will show a more protracted diminished sensitivity to blood oxygen levels because it retains the foetal ventilation response to rising carbon dioxide levels rather than oxygen.

In the first two to twelve weeks of extra-uterine life, the muscles in the pulmonary arteries become thinner, dilate, lengthen and branch, which further reduces the resistance of the pulmonary vasculature and pressure of blood in the right side of the heart. However, the anatomy is still very reactive to hypoxia, acidosis, over-distension of the alveoli and hypothermia. Over the next one to two months, the pulmonary vessels gradually function as in the adult, and throughout childhood the arteries develop better muscle in those supplying the bronchi, bronchioles and alveoli. Local cyanosis of trunk and extremities can result from venous stasis and vascular instability in young children, often associated with low ambient temperature, and is not a sign of decreased oxygen saturation (Chandler 2000). Infants up to four weeks are obligatory nose breathers – thus the risk to their breathing increases if they have colds or lie with their face in vomit or bedding (www.clinicalevidence.com, www.fsid.org.uk). They adapt later to mouth breathing. They have small airways which will narrow further if swollen or blocked with secretions; they have to work harder to breathe against this increased resistance. Young babies who have difficulty with breathing will also have difficulty feeding and soon lose weight (see Chapter 7 on the digestive system). Airway resistance in all children is higher than the adult due to the smaller diameter of tubes throughout their respiratory system.

The patency of the upper airways is maintained by the active contraction of muscles in the pharynx and larynx. These muscles, if compromised when the neck is flexed or extended, will lead to the airway being compromised. The glottis, which is the entrance to the trachea, lies higher in the throat than in that of the adult, there is more cephalid in the infant than the five-year-old, the laryngeal reflexes are more active and the epiglottis is longer. This will have importance if resuscitation is performed; the head position for artificial resuscitation aims to open the airway for re-breathing – the 'sniffing position' is thus recommended for small children under five years of age (see resuscitation advice section).

There is areolar tissue present below the vocal cords in the larynx of young children which is not evident in the adult; this will swell and block the tracheal lumen if inflamed or traumatised such as when the child suffers croup or persistent coughing. The narrowest part of the airway in the child is at the lower level of the larynx, the cricoid cartilage, whereas in the adult it is higher. Vocal cords vibrate when air passes through them; children have slender, short vocal cords and thus their voices tend to be high-pitched. At puberty, the larynx of a male will enlarge more than that of the female under the influence of rising testosterone levels in the blood, and the vocal cords will become thicker and stronger and thus produce lower voice tones of the adult male.

The trachea is also very elastic and flexible in the infant. Babies have high tracheal bifurcation to the bronchi at the third thoracic vertebral level: important anatomical knowledge for tracheal suctioning. They need their heads supported at all times when handling them and when placing them in the horizontal position the jaw at right angles to the spine to avoid compromising their airways.

The upper respiratory tract is short; the risk of infective material entering is high. Small babies are susceptible to droplet spread of viruses and bacteria, for example colds and meningitis. The air sacs are not complete in number, and there is a relatively small area for gas exchange: if occluded by mucus and exudate the gas exchange reduces further. The round thoracic capacity, resulting from ribs lying horizontally and weak intercostal muscles, results in the diaphragm and abdomen being the primary means of ventilation (Marieb and Hoehn 2007). The diaphragm, serviced by the phrenic nerve, cannot contract as much or as effectively as in the older child because it is attached higher at the front of the chest and thus is relatively longer and is not fully enervated so more prone to fatigue (Aylott 2006).

The small child's breathing

When a small child makes respiratory effort the chest wall is more compliant (stretchy) than the adult, because only the external intercostal muscles, which elevate the ribs for inspiration, stabilise the chest wall. The diaphragm is more horizontal and there is lower rib retraction when the child lies supine. The greater the rib retraction the more the diaphragm will need to contract to generate tidal volume; this is a very inefficient way to breathe and the muscles will tire quickly when ventilation is increased for long periods. Small children will display a chest wall that deforms inwards, nasal flaring, grunting breathing, open mouth in inspiration and pursed lips in expiration when they experience breathing difficulties; they use a lot of energy and become fatigued quickly. Heat and water are transmitted from the respiratory tract to expired air; children lose relatively more body heat and water from their body tissues in breathing, so are more likely to develop sticky mucus plugs when they have respiratory infections.

Airways increase in length and diameter after birth. Until three years, the number of immature alveoli increases; after this age the size only increases. Blood vessels continue to be remodelled and increase in number as the new alveoli are forming. These 'terminal units' increase in size and number until the child reaches the age of eight years. Also, alveoli and bronchiole pathways for collateral ventilation (pores to allow trapped gas in obstructed airways to be absorbed) continue to develop until this age.

Apnoea

This is a period of breathing absence lasting twenty seconds or more, or a shorter time if the child develops a bluish or pale colour or the heart rate drops. Many infants have periods of rapid breathing alternating with periods of slow rate, or they may not breathe for periods up to fifteen seconds. This is normal if the colour and heart rate do not change considerably and the infant starts to breathe spontaneously. True apnoea is only common in premature infants below thirty-two weeks. It can be reduced in the neonatal unit by minimal handling, keeping the infant's temperature constant and placing the infant in the prone position. Medically, they can be treated with caffeine which quickly stimulates the medulla and pons, the central nervous controls of respiration.

Apnoea is caused by respiratory, central nervous system, metabolic and obstructive abnormalities. Common causes are when the child is exhausted, has pneumonia or a pneumothorax, has aspirated some solid or fluid, or has had the vagus nerve stimulated in the pharynx such as when passing a naso-gastric feeding tube or over-suctioning the pharynx/trachea. Central causes of apnoea in children are due to an immature/underdeveloped respiratory control centre or when they have a seizure. Seizures can occur unexpectedly in hyperpyrexia (often a temperature in excess of 40 °C), and are most often seen in children under five years of age whose temperature control mechanisms in the hypothalamus are immature. Central nervous system abnormalities such as cerebral haemorrhage, cerebral birth trauma, kernicterus and meningitis are all rarer stimuli for apnoea, but breathing absence may be their first symptom if the medulla and pons are involved. Metabolic effects of mineral deficiencies, low blood sugar and drug therapy can also quickly affect the body systems' homeostatic balance which may subsequently influence ventilation stimuli from the brain. Congenital and secondary obstruction, such as anatomical airway obstruction at birth or the child's face being covered at any age, also result in cessation of ventilation and thus oxygenation of body tissues.

Respiratory resuscitation

This may be required as an emergency procedure and if the child is choking. Procedures are based on the Resuscitation Council (UK) guidelines (www.resus.org.uk). Health and social professionals, such as doctors and nurses (a first aider is not a health care professional) who would normally not resuscitate infants and children in the course of their work, should normally use the adult sequence of procedures with paediatric modifiers. Child minders, parents and 'early years' workers should all be taught adult resuscitation with paediatric modifiers. Full details of all procedures are updated and freely available on the Resuscitation Council website (see above).

Paediatric 'modifiers' to adult resuscitation procedure:

- give five initial breaths before starting chest compression;
- if on your own, perform one minute CPR (cardio-pulmonary-resuscitation) before going for help;
- compress the chest approximately one-third of its depth. Use two fingers for an infant under one year; use one or two hands for a child over one year as needed to achieve an adequate depth of compression.

Changes at puberty

From five years to puberty the weight of the lungs increases threefold, vital capacity rises from 1,000 to 3,000 cc, and total lung capacity improves from 1,400 to 4,500 cc in the child on the 50 per cent percentile (see Chapter 10 for an explanation of percentile). Resting total lung volume increases as the lungs grow; this change is seen equally in boys and in girls. Respiratory rates tend to be slightly higher in boys, perhaps due to their changing lean body mass as they approach puberty and their increase in lean muscle tissue which has a higher metabolic demand for oxygen than fat. Maturation of the respiratory system tissues is complete by eight years. From eight years and through puberty, increased air space occurs through enlargement of the alveoli and airways. Throughout childhood the volume of the lungs remains at a constant ratio to body mass; lung capacity correlates best with the changing body height. Ventilation, duration of inspiration and expiration are all influenced by resistance to flow in the airways and the elasticity (compliance) of the lung tissue. Resistance is created by friction of flow within both the lung and the upper airways. Smoking cigarettes and living in a polluted air environment in this period will damage the fragile respiratory tract linings and the developing air sacs. Compliance is determined by the elastic properties of the lung, connective tissues and the alveolar surface forces, as well as the chest wall. As the child grows and the airways enlarge, resistance reduces and respiration rate decreases (Table 5.1). Compliance, which has improved most rapidly in the first two years and remained relatively high until five years, now increases faster than resistance declines. Arets (2007) found that children aged four to twelve who lived with parents who smoked had significantly reduced lung function similar to that seen in smokers; he suggested that smoking restrictions imposed for public places may put children further at risk as parents are forced to smoke more in their own homes. Gauderman *et al.* (2007) showed that children living near motorways are more likely to develop asthma and other respiratory diseases and showed lower volume lung development than those who lived away from traffic congested areas.

Table 5.1 Respiratory rates in children

Age	*Rate*	*Too high*
Newborn	30–50	Over 60
1 year	26–40	Over 50
2 years	20–30	
4 years	20–26	Over 40
5 years	19–25	
6 years	18–24	
7 years	17–24	
8 years	17–23	
9 years	16–23	
10 years	15–22	
11 years	14–21	
12 years	14–21	
13 years	13–20	
14 years	12–20	
15 years	12–19	
16 years	11–14	

Source: Adapted from Wallis *et al.* (2005) for children at rest in the 2.5–97.5 centile range.

Note: Rates may be higher by 10 per cent if the child is awake, anxious or restless (Aylott 2006).

Measuring respiratory rates

It must be remembered that the assessment of respiration depends on the child's cooperation and should be measured for a complete minute when the child is at rest (Aylott 2006). Most of resting inspiration is due to diaphragmatic contraction so there is little apparent chest movement; in normal respiration, the child's chest and abdomen move out together. Peak expiratory flow (PEF) is a simple test of lung function: the highest flow achieved from a maximal forced expiratory manoeuvre started without hesitation from a position of maximal lung inflation (Tantucci *et al.* 2002). It is measured in litres per minute and occurs in the first tenth of a second of the expiration. Children under the age of six years are unreliable with their technique, such as not making maximal effort in the three readings required, so PEF is not useful for the younger child (Booker 2007). Measured effort will be related to their ability to coordinate breathing and blowing into the apparatus. Small children also have difficulty conforming to requests for measurement due to their immature central synchronisation controls and weaker muscle function and they often fear masks and restraint. Boran *et al.* (2007) investigated respiratory resistance in obese children but found that mild obesity effects were minimal; however, gross obesity will restrict chest movement on exertion. Reference values for the normal range of lung function are related to height alone for children, whereas in the adult they are related to age, gender and height combinations. Thus, when prescribing inhalers and monitoring for asthma, a common respiratory condition in childhood, children must have age-related apparatus for their use and their lung function must be assessed in relation to their height.

Respiration during exercise

Exercise increases demand for oxygen by the muscle cells and excretion of carbon dioxide; this leads to increased alveolar ventilation, increased cardiac output and redistribution of blood to muscles. These three physiological functions are changing as the child grows and matures, and respond to the physical nature of the lifestyle they experience. While the child can provide oxygen to the muscle cells for energy production, complete breakdown of the sugar molecule takes place to release ATP (cell energy), and carbon dioxide and water are the waste products (aerobic respiration). If oxygen levels fall, anaerobic respiration takes place in the muscle cells for a short period of time where lactic acid is produced from the incomplete breakdown of glucose to release ATP; this may cause a burning sensation in the muscle. The blood transports the lactic acid eventually from the muscles to the liver where oxygen is used to convert it back to glucose. The child may continue to breathe heavily after strenuous exercise as it pays an 'oxygen debt' (Thibodeau and Patton 2007). Overall ventilation can increase twenty-fold in exercise; it increases as the strength and rate of contraction of the respiratory muscles increases. Blood flow to the respiratory muscles increases by 5 to 12 per cent. In the lungs, perfusion of the pulmonary capillaries increases as oxygen is drawn into the alveoli. There is a raised oxygen extraction by muscles as temperature rises and acidity of the blood falls due to carbon dioxide excretion; oxygen unloading from the blood to the cells also speeds up as more carbon dioxide that is made from glucose breakdown is 'exchanged' with oxygen.

Young people appear to have a more favourable peripheral distribution of blood during exercise, which facilitates the transport of oxygen to the exercising muscles. Children appear to have slightly more mitochondria and an elevated level of some enzymes that aid oxygen use by the cells in their body tissue cells when compared to adults, perhaps increasing the oxidative capacity of their muscles. However, they have significantly lower muscle cell glycogen stores (stored energy) than adults and they appear to be less able than adults to generate ATP (adenosine triphosphate – the cell energy source) via glycogen breakdown when performing strenuous (anaerobic) exercise for excess of periods of ten to sixty seconds. Anaerobic performance increases with age; boys of eight years have only 70 per cent performance compared to boys of eleven years who have bigger muscles. Girls show a constant improvement of muscle function with age; they peak in their teen years but never achieve the performance of boys, whose anaerobic capacity increases further as they mature through puberty.

Children hyperventilate during exercise, their patterns of ventilation changing as they grow. It may be due to age-related differences in lung size, neural controls or to the size-related differences in the ventilation mechanisms. It may also be due to their changing lung compliance and airway resistance. Children have changing lean/fat ratios as they move through childhood, and this will affect gas uptake because carbon dioxide will be stored in their fat tissue. They have lower haemoglobin concentrations than adults; in gas exchange haemoglobin binds carbon dioxide and acts as a buffer to hydrogen ions in the blood where this gas is dissolved and carried as carbonic acid. Over long periods of aerobic activity, they are disadvantaged because, although their oxygen uptake is at least as good as adults, they have smaller stores of muscle glycogen and immature temperature regulation systems. Formal exercise, such as physical training programmes, during childhood must be approached with caution, especially if the environment conditions are adverse.

During maximal exercise a five-year-old may have a minute volume of 35 L, whereas an adult may reach 150 L or more; minute volume being the amount of air moved by the lungs per minute. Children have shallower and more frequent breathing rates but, related to body mass, they have the same minute volume as adults. At any level of exercise smaller children breathe more to deliver a given amount of oxygen to their blood, and thus to their body cells, than do adolescents. Smaller children also appear to have a ventilation drive more sensitive to carbon dioxide. As it is alveoli ventilation that drives gas exchange, and children have a smaller 'dead space' than adults, their alveoli ventilation is adequate for exercise (Armstrong 2007). The sex difference between children's peak oxygen values in exercise, their aerobic fitness, can be attributed to habitual physical activity and haemoglobin concentration. Boys have been consistently shown to be more physically active than girls and show a greater percentage of lean body mass. Interestingly, boys also show higher oxygen uptake even though their haemoglobin is similar to girls in the pre-pubertal years.

At puberty, however, the differences between the sexes are evident as boys develop a greater muscle mass and higher haemoglobin concentration under the effect of testosterone. Boys' maximal oxygen uptake increases by about 150 per cent over the age range eight to sixteen years, with girls demonstrating only an 80 per cent increase. Boys' values are about 13 per cent higher than girls at the age of ten years, with an increase to 37 per cent at sixteen years. However, in twelve- to sixteen-year-old males, body mass, age and height explain 74 per cent of the variance; serum testosterone did not significantly raise the scores. In girls, the accumulation of body fat in the pubertal years reduced their maximal oxygen uptake, whereas boys in the age range ten to sixteen years remained consistent to mass, age and height. Research continues on the effect of maturation on exercise performance of respiratory function in older children, and how exercise can improve peripheral oxygen extraction in the developing cardiovascular system and muscles.

Breathing changes during sleep

We spend 30 per cent of our lives asleep. In REM, or deep sleep, respiration is regular and ventilation reduces in relation to the reduced metabolic demand. Slowing of respiratory rate occurs as the child slips into the deep sleep state. The parasympathetic nerve supply dominates regulation of airway function; the bronchi/bronchiole muscles relax and reduce their lumen size. It is this action that can stimulate a child to wake, feel breathless and cough if their bronchial airways are irritated; commonly seen when children suffer from chronic airway conditions such as asthma. In REM sleep, where dreaming occurs, respiration becomes irregular and the respiratory muscle activity is altered. Tonic intercostal muscle activity is partly abolished and rhythmic activity is reduced; phasic diaphragm activity compensates. There is a small decrease in ventilatory response to hypoxia, and loss of the tonic and inspiratory phase is also linked to relaxing of the throat muscles. Tidal volume, the amount of air moved in one inspiration, reduces. In healthy children's sleep, true apnoea is uncommon, however, short (less than ten second) periods of central cyanosis can be seen during REM sleep but reduction of oxygen levels is not usually apparent (Uliel *et al.* 2004). Small babies have longer REM sleep periods so are regularly seen to have irregular breathing and oscillation movement of eyeballs under their eyelids as they dream. Any swelling of their upper airway will compromise their oxygen intake as the throat and soft palate muscles relax and the tongue falls back in the pharynx. A child in respiratory distress will become cyanotic (look pale with a blue tinge round their nose and mouth), have nasal flaring, grunt and demonstrate retraction of tissue around the throat and chest. In the assessment of the child's respiratory system, the brain and central nervous system control, airway, chest wall, respiratory muscles and lung tissue all need to be considered.

Development of the ear

In the upper respiratory tract, air enters the trachea via the nose and throat. The ear is closely connected to these passages by the Eustachian tube which is composed partly of bone and partly of cartilage and fibrous tissue and lined with mucosa. It extends from the middle ear to the nasopharynx (the part of the throat behind the nose) and allows equalisation of pressure either side of the tympanic membrane to avoid its rupture (Thibodeau and Patton 2007). This can be demonstrated by swallowing or yawning when pressure changes are experienced in aeroplane cabins at take off and landing.

The inner ear develops at each side of the hindbrain at four weeks' gestation, and the middle ear starts to develop from the first pharyngeal pouch at this time. The external ear then develops from the first and second branchial grooves and, until the twenty-eighth week of gestation, remains plugged with epithelial cells which will normally disperse before birth. Rubella virus contracted by the mother in the first trimester of pregnancy results in damage to the inner ear because the seventh week is a critical time for its formation. Debate within the profession on the danger of early sonar scanning of the pregnant woman in relation to ear damage in the foetus is interesting from this development point of view.

At birth the infant reacts to sound, of which the human voice is preferred; startle and blink reflexes occur at sudden noise. At one month, the infant notices prolonged sounds such as a vacuum cleaner noise. At four months it will turn the head to voices and will quieten to familiar sounds and will turn to a noise source from some distance by seven months. At nine months it will listen attentively and show pleasure in babbling, and should by one year respond to familiar words.

To examine the ear of a child, the appropriate size of equipment is necessary, together with an understanding of the anatomical changes that take place over childhood. The lobe of the infant ear should be moved down and back to straighten the upward-curving ear canal in order to visualise the tympanic membrane. In children over three years the canal curves downward and forward, thus the ear lobe needs to be gently pulled up and back.

Discussion about insertion of grommets surrounds the evidence that some children improve spontaneously from chronic infection of these tiny airways, yet others suffer hearing loss as great as fifty decibels. Few children escape some symptoms of secretory otitis media (glue ear) in childhood, as upper respiratory infections of the throat, nose and ear are common at this time. The anatomy of the young child's upper respiratory tract is small and structures are relatively close together, thus infections such as the common cold causing inflammation of the lining mucosa in the nasal passages and pharynx will soon involve other associated structures in the ear (NHS Direct website, www.nhsdirect.nhs.uk). There is indication that passive smoking also puts children at risk because inhaled cigarette smoke impairs the mucocillary function in these nasopharyngeal tissues, causing an inflammatory exudate that blocks the tiny tubes. When feeding fluids to an infant or toddler, a semi-prone position is recommended, as they are less likely to experience reflux of milk into the narrow Eustachian tube (Figures 5.3 and 5.4). The use of feeding cups in bed for the older child may also encourage the development of glue ear and recurrent middle ear infections.

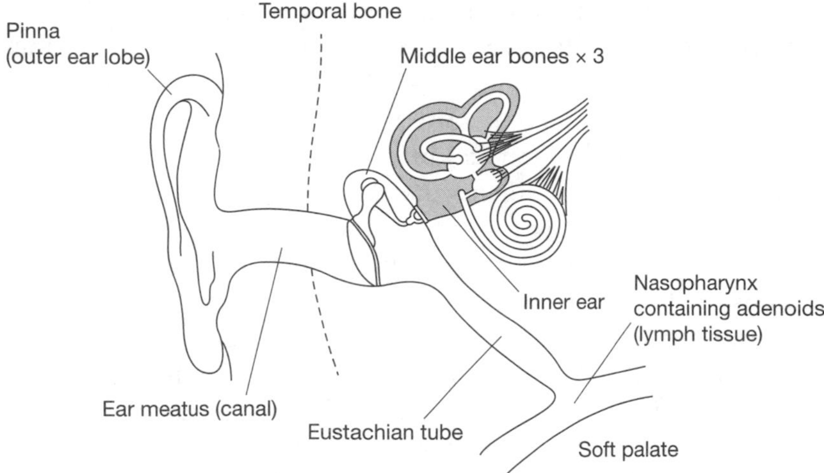

Figure 5.3 The Eustachian tube's position

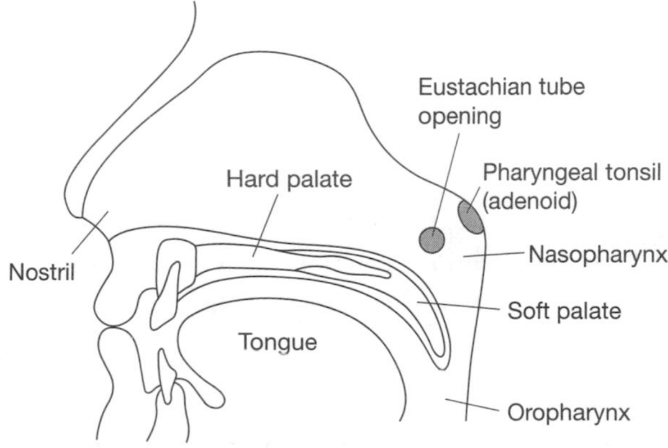

Figure 5.4 The Eustachian tube opening in the nasopharynx

Physiology knowledge in practice

Scenario 1

Twins Mary and Sam, aged ten years, have lived in a house which fronts onto the main high street of a rural town all their lives. Traffic is heavy twenty-four hours a day, seven days a week. What could be the affect on the children's lung development in experiencing constant air pollution from passing traffic 24/7?

Some pointers:

- Lung growth may have been stunted. This can be measured by reduced peak flow recordings for their age – a lower force and volume of air expired in the first second of each breath. This will reduce their overall breathing capacity in adult life and put them at risk of chronic airway diseases (Gauderman *et al.* 2007). Note to reader for revision of knowledge: Revise structure of the alveoli and how gas exchange takes place.
- Lung development and maturation continue throughout childhood, the main growth period being in the under eight group.
- They may already suffer from asthma and/or recurrent chest infections or decreased capacity for physical exercise. They may not enjoy sports or leisure activities where their breathing is challenged and thus will miss other opportunities to exercise their lungs. This may result in their choosing sedentary occupations in their free time or remaining at home when they are sick rather than socialising with their peer group.
- The fine carbon emissions will have damaged the lining mucosa of the respiratory system where protective fluid and white cell phagocytes protect the tissues.

Scenario 2

Sally, aged fifteen years, continues to breathe deeply on completing a 100-m race at her school sports day. What is the physiological reason in relation to her respiratory system?

The theory

- In exercise the muscles use oxygen more rapidly than at rest; they require more oxygen and glucose to release energy for work.

- One waste product of glucose metabolism is carbon dioxide. This gas is released from the body cells into the blood and is carried to the lungs as carbonic acid. The blood thus becomes more acid as more glucose is broken down to release energy and stimulates the chemoreceptors in the medulla (respiratory centre) in the brain.
- The medulla responds by increasing ventilation of the lungs to expel carbon dioxide and take in more oxygen. It does this by stimulating the intercostal muscles and diaphragm to increase and deepen the respiratory rate.
- When the exercise stops the oxygen debt must be completely repaid in order for the cells to metabolise lactic acid, which was formed in the muscles after breakdown of glucose when little oxygen was present. Sally will continue to breathe heavily until this is done.
- Sally may not run fast regularly so her ability to transfer oxygen to her muscle cells may be slower than her more athletic peers. Her intercostal muscles may also be tired after her run and her heavy breathing, as she repays her oxygen debt, may take longer than usual to return to normal.
- There are many other aspects of this incident that may affect Sally's experience and subsequent recovery. You might like to consider her cardiovascular system and temperature control separately for yourself.

Extend your knowledge

The American Academy of Otolarygology – Head and Neck Surgery has a public education campaign website (www.entnet.org). In 2006 they reported that 17:1,000 children under the age of eighteen had some sort of hearing loss. Access this web page and consider your views on the increase of dangerous noise levels that may affect children's hearing such as TV, music speakers and iPods. What could be done about the risk to children's hearing and what might be the consequences for them if noise levels continue to rise.

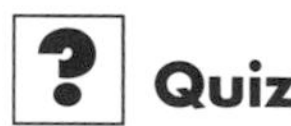

Quiz

1 What changes in respiration can be seen over the first week of an infant's life?

2 What structure does the lung bud develop from in embryonic development?
3 Why is foetal lung resistance high?
4 When does surfactant secretion start in the lung?
5 How does surfactant work?
6 What stimulates a term infant to take its first breath?
7 What is the risk to the neonate of having its nose occluded?
8 What is the difference in the structure of the larynx between boys and girls?
9 What is the difference in a child breathing in comparison to an adult?
10 What is apnoea?
11 What are the paediatric modifiers for child resuscitation?
12 Why are respiratory rates usually higher in pubescent boys than pubescent girls?
13 What does lung compliance mean?
14 What is the average respiratory rate of a four-year-old and what measurement would inform you that a child of this age is breathing too fast?
15 What is PEF?
16 Why are children not able to exercise as efficiently as adults?
17 What happens to the respiratory airways in deep sleep?
18 How does respiration change when children dream?
19 How is the ear connected to the airways?
20 Why do upper respiratory tract infections often lead to ear symptoms in young children?

Further reading

Wallis, L.A. and Maconochie, I. (2006) 'Age-related reference ranges of respiratory and heart rate for children in South Africa', *Archives of Diseases in Children*, 91(4): 330–333.

www.besttreatments.co.uk, accessed July 2007

Chapter 6

The renal system

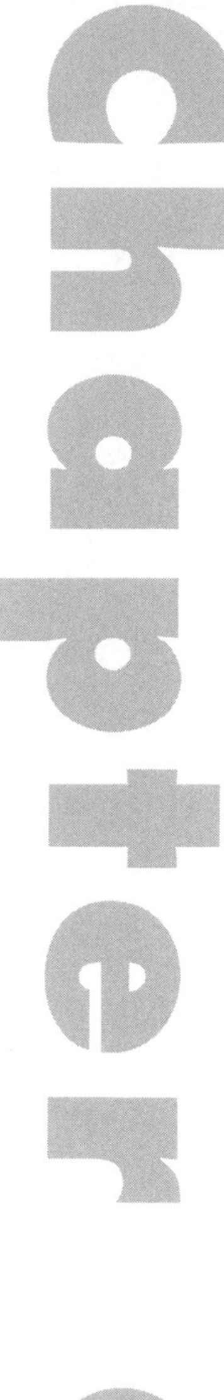

- Water balance
- Embryo urinary system development
- The kidney and urine production at birth
- Fluid requirements in the first week
- Developing continence
- Bed wetting – nocturnal enuresis
- Gaining continence
- Dehydration and rehydration
- Urine

THE RENAL (URINARY SYSTEM) consists of two kidneys, one urinary bladder and one urethra. The kidneys constantly filter the blood plasma (filtrate) through capillary networks called glomeruli and return most of the water and solutes back to the blood throughout the tiny filtering tubules called nephrons (see Figure 6.1). The waste products are excreted as urine, which consists of the excess water and solutes together with other wastes such as urea (a toxin to body cells), that is made from the breakdown of proteins and bilirubin (which gives urine its yellow colour) produced from the breakdown of red blood cell haemoglobin. The kidneys regulate blood minerals such as sodium and potassium, blood acidity within the normal pH 7.35–7.45 range and vascular pressure. They also produce two hormones: calcitol, which is activated vitamin D, that allows absorption of calcium from the gut for bone development; and erythropoietin, which stimulates the bone marrow to manufacture red blood cells when blood oxygen carrying capacity becomes low (Marieb and Hoehn 2007). The renal system is critical to the healthy function of all body systems.

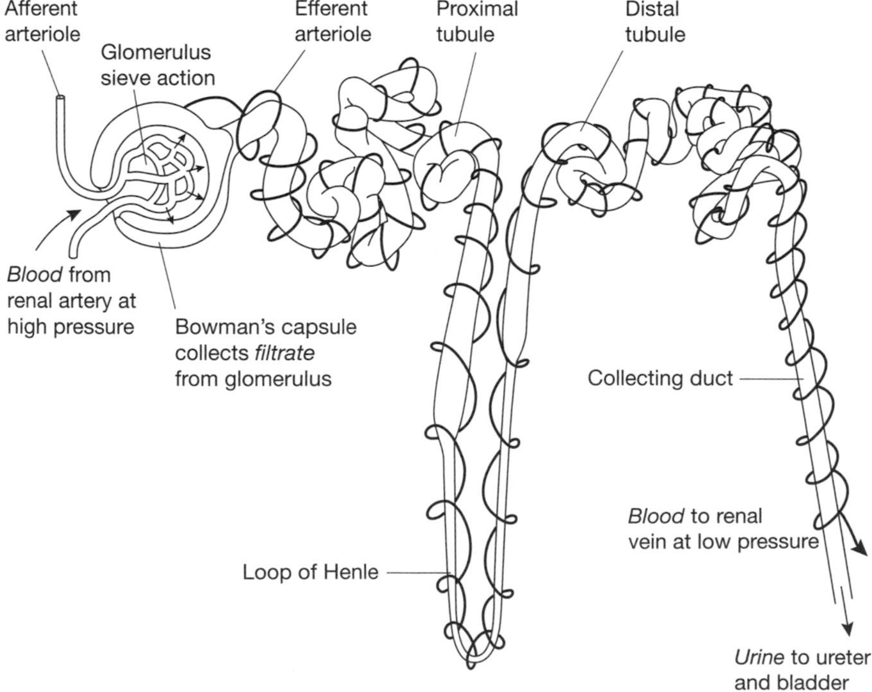

Figure 6.1 The filtering agent of the kidney – the nephron

Water balance

Intake and output of water (water balance) is vital to all living organisms; body water is the largest component of body tissues, comprising 70 per cent in the infant and decreasing over childhood to 60 per cent in the adult. Water is mainly present in two 'compartments'; two thirds in the intracellular spaces and one third in the extra cellular spaces (80 per cent of this in the interstitial spaces and 20 per cent in the plasma). There are other pockets of fluid also in many other parts of the body serving vital functions; this 'third compartment' consists of fluids such as the lymph fluid, cerebral spinal fluid, parts of the eye and ear, fluid in the pleural, pericardial and peritoneal cavities (McCance and Heuther 2006). In the child there is a higher amount of the water outside the cells in the interstitial spaces, and there is a higher turnover of water due to an immature kidney function to conserve water. Young children also have a larger surface area:volume ratio and are therefore vulnerable to excess water loss from breathing and sweating to the outside environment – such as when they take part in physical play on a hot day. They have a larger circulating blood volume per kilogram of body weight, but their overall volume is small, so loss of blood volume in haemorrhage has a more devastating effect and quickly affects the function of all vital body organs. Children take in water from their diet, normally controlled automatically by their sensation of thirst, a dry mouth and the hypothalamus thirst centre stimulus. They need to be offered regular drinks as they are often 'too busy' to ask. They also produce more water as a by-product of their high metabolic rate. They lose water mainly through their larger skin surface to body mass, their relatively longer gut and their more rapid breathing. Diarrhoea and vomiting are important symptoms to address when children are ill because they can not afford to lose water this way. Table 6.1 overleaf shows daily fluid requirements for children of different ages.

Most babies lose weight in the first few days after birth. This drop is normally less than 10 per cent of the birth weight. Physiological weight loss is the result of fluid loss by evaporation from the skin, micturition, defecation and respiratory exchange. The first urine to be passed is colourless and odourless, with a specific gravity of 1.020 (London *et al.* 2007).

Table 6.1 Daily average fluid requirements for children calculated by body weight

Age	*Body weight in kg*	*Water (ml/kg/24 hours)*
Newborn	3	80–100
1 year	9.5	120–135
4 years	16.2	100–110
10 years	28.7	70–85
14 years	45	50–60

The total water content of an infant's body is vulnerable to loss because they ingest and excrete a relatively greater water volume each day. An infant may exchange half of his or her extra-cellular fluid (ECF) daily, whereas the adult may only exchange one-sixth; so proportionally the baby has less reserve of body fluid at any one time. This is also due to their metabolic rate which is twice that of adults per unit of body weight; infants expend 100 kcal/kg of body weight, whereas adults expend 40 kcal/kg, they thus expel more body waste due to their high metabolic rate, so their kidneys need to form a large volume of fluid for this activity.

Throughout childhood, total body fluids reduce towards adult levels. By puberty, the adult composition is attained and also shows a sex difference. Fat tissue contains little water; muscle tissue contains more; females, with relatively more body fat due to the effect of oestrogen in puberty increasing fat deposits, have less total body fluid than males and any obese child, female or male, has less than their lean peers.

Embryo urinary system development

Knowledge of the development of the urinary tract will enable the reader to understand how abnormalities can easily occur while the foetus is growing and why young babies have difficulties with fluid challenges. The system develops from the intermediate mesoderm on either side of the dorsal (back) body wall, which gives rise to three successive nephric structures (filtering units) of increasingly advanced design. The kidney changes three times before it is completed! The first kidneys are transitory, non-functional segmental nephrotomes in the cranial region which regress in the fourth week on day twenty-four to twenty-five. After this, an elongated pair of mesonephroi appear in the thoracic and lumbar region either side of the vertebral column. These structures are functional, as they have complete nephrons and drain caudally via the Wolffian ducts to the urogenital sinus. By week five the ureteric buds (Figure 6.2) sprout from the Wolffian ducts and develop into the definitive kidneys that will serve the child for life (Chamley *et al.* 2005).

The bladder expands from the superior urogenic sinus and the inferior section gives rise to the urethra in both sexes. Ureters are then emplaced on the bladder wall. This articulation can give rise to multiple ureters forming or joining with the bladder ineffectively. At week six, germ cells migrating from the yolk sac induce the mesonephros to differentiate into Sertoli cells in the male and follicle cells in the female (see Chapter 8 on the reproductive system). At the same time a new Müllerian duct develops parallel to the mesonephric duct. It is in week six, when the Y chromosome exerts its effect, that a development cascade then sees the forming of the male or female external genitalia and the kidneys ascending to their lumbar site in the abdomen, the right being lower than the left due to the presence of the liver.

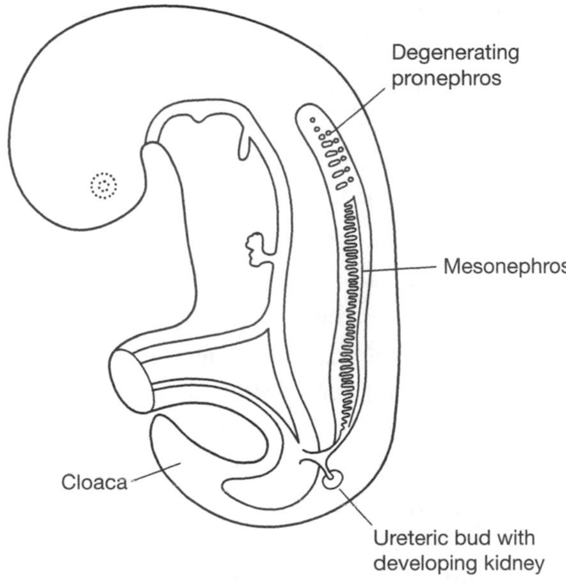

Figure 6.2 Kidney bud position

By the tenth week, the foetal kidney is functional and commences urine production. Foetal urine is important, not to get rid of waste products from the blood as the placenta regulates fluid and electrolyte homeostasis, but to supplement the production of amniotic fluid. Amniotic fluid is vital to the foetal development as it contains proteins, carbohydrates, lipids and phospholipids, urea and electrolytes. It is a clear slightly yellow liquid round the foetus and increases during the pregnancy to 800 ml at thirty-four weeks. It is constantly circulated by the foetus as it swallows and 'inhales' the fluid, replacing it by 'exhalation' and urination. The amniotic fluid protects the foetus by cushioning it from outside crushing, allows it to move and develop its muscular-skeletal system, keeps it at an even temperature and allows the lungs and gut to mature (see www.nlm.nih.gov/medlineplus/ency/article00220).

The kidney and urine production at birth

The neonate has an immature kidney function at birth which makes it vulnerable to water loss and fluid gain, such as losing fluid through rapid breathing or failure to feed. The neonate's kidneys weigh about 23 g but have their full complement of filtering units (nephrons); this weight will double in six months and treble by the end of the first year eventually growing to its adult size by puberty which shows a ten-fold increase from birth. The growth of the kidney depends on its work; if one kidney is removed the other will double in size and take on the function of both.

When the infant is born the loss of placenta flow, followed by a rapid increase in the infant's own renal blood flow, causes a high vascular resistance in the neonate kidney. This results in a temporarily reduced renal blood flow and filtration through the filtering units to produce urine; however, as the infant starts to feed and the load presented to the kidney increases, 95 per cent of infants will pass urine in the first twenty-four hours after birth. The neonate will pass 20–35 ml of urine four times a day while intake is low and milk production establishes in the mother, but this soon rises to 100–200 ml ten times a day by the tenth day of life. The urine that is first produced shows reduced urea excretion because of the overall tissue growth rate in the infant that uses the protein rather than allowing it to be broken down in the liver. Also, in the first few days, urea is deposited in the kidney medulla to create the concentration gradient for the Loop of Henle function in adjusting water and sodium in the blood. Growth is thus sometimes referred to as the 'third kidney'.

The kidney capillary network resistance reduces over the first few weeks of life, which allows increasing filtration ability by the glomeruli, however, the newborn kidney glomeruli capsules are formed of cuboid epithelium and are not fully replaced by thin pavement epithelium and fully functional until after the first year. These small, immature nephrons also have short Loops of Henle where water and sodium are normally adjusted; salt (sodium) should not be added to an infant's diet as it cannot excrete the excess to requirements easily and the excess sodium will retain water in the arteries and veins, raise blood pressure and dilate the developing heart (Table 6.2). The infant's distal convoluted tubules in the nephron are relatively resistant to the hormone aldosterone, released from the adrenal cortex in response to high blood sodium, which results in limited excretion of sodium and thus concentrating ability of urine in the infant. A reduced glomerulus filtration rate (GFR) 28–30 ml/min/m^2 at birth increases over time to approximately 100 ml/min/m^2 at nine months, and reaching 30 to 50 per cent of adult values at one to two years (McCance and Heuther 2006).

Difficulty in excretion of acids impairs the ability of the kidney to correct acidosis – for example, if the infant is underfed it will breakdown body fat for energy (ketones are released as a waste product in fat breakdown which reduces the blood pH acidity and may irritate the brain). The infant blood pH average is slightly lower (more acidic) than the older child at 7.3–7.35 (normal range 7.35–7.45) thus the blood acidity will fall more quickly the younger the child and body responses will occur more rapidly.

Table 6.2 Normal venous blood electrolyte values

Component	*Amount (mmols/l)*
Sodium	135–145
Potassium	3.5–4.5
Urea	2.5–4.5
Phosphate	0.8–1.4
Creatinine	0–6

Source: Glasper *et al.* 2007.

Fluid requirements in the first week

Fluid requirements, ml/kg/24 hours, increase with weight (Table 6.3). Milk intake appears to be highly individual, as is the timing, but a guide is often useful for the new mother. They should not over or under-feed their babies from ignorance (see Chapter 7 on the digestive system). Young babies need to feed little and often, whereas older babies can take larger amounts of fluid less often because their stomach volume is larger. Fluid intake also has to be adjusted for ambient temperatures and the condition of the baby. The newborn infant has a surface area relatively two to three times that of the adult, thus a greater proportion of water will be lost through insensible routes such as through the skin and during increased breathing rates; dehydration occurs more rapidly the smaller the child.

Developing continence

Infants are expected to be incontinent, but the ability to control voiding of urine depends on a complete and functioning renal system, maturation of the nervous supply, opportunity/support given to the child to void and cultural expectations. Children can become anxious and regress if expectations are beyond their ability and control. The maturation of control mechanisms usually takes up to five years for healthy children to be dry in the day and overnight. The urinary bladder is a complex organ made of specialised muscle layers and enervated by a reflex arc to the spine and central coordination in the brain. Remember that if the child does not want to void, for whatever reason, they can override the messages to their brain from their distending bladder.

Table 6.3 Feed requirements (ml)

Day 1	30
Day 2	60
Day 3	90
Day 4	120
Day 5	150

Source: Glasper *et al.* 2007.

In the infant, the urinary bladder is an abdominal organ descending into the pelvis as more space becomes available. It is formed of four layers. The inner mucosa is folded into rugae and connected to the muscle layer by connective tissue. The bladder muscle, detrusor, is a sandwich of circular muscle between two layers of longitudinal muscle. The lower posterior wall is called the trigone, a triangular area where there are a large number of stretch receptors which respond to bladder filling. The base of the bladder neck joins to the urethra and here are the urinary sphincter mechanisms. At the neck of the bladder is a ring of smooth muscle, circular in the male and longitudinal in females, the internal sphincter. Below this, made of both smooth and striated muscle, lies the external sphincter. These are normally kept closed by the pelvic floor striated muscle (Figure 6.3).

The ability to control bladder emptying is a process that is learnt usually in early childhood as a result of 'potty training'. A baby is incapable of exercising any control over this process, because bladder emptying is dependent on the action of the reflex arc (Figure 6.4). Their bladder will voluntarily empty when stretched by a volume of 15 ml, whereas the adult stimulus to void is a volume of 200 ml. When the bladder fills it distends the trigone stretch receptors, and these in turn send impulses to the sacral area of the spine via the autonomic nervous system. Motor impulses from the spinal cord via the autonomic nervous system initiate relaxation of the internal sphincter and contraction of the detrusor muscle, leading to urine

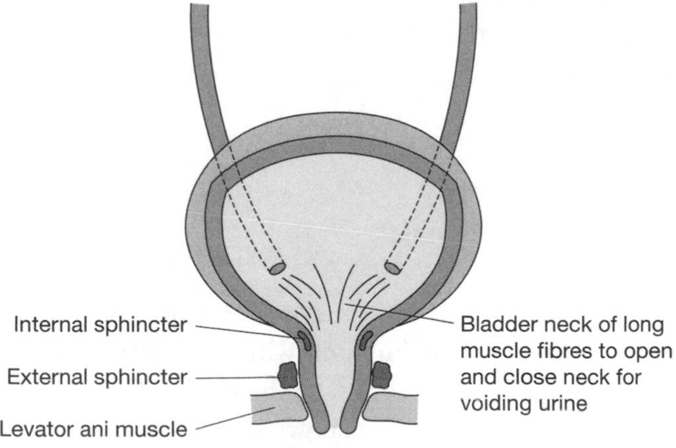

Figure 6.3 Bladder sphincters

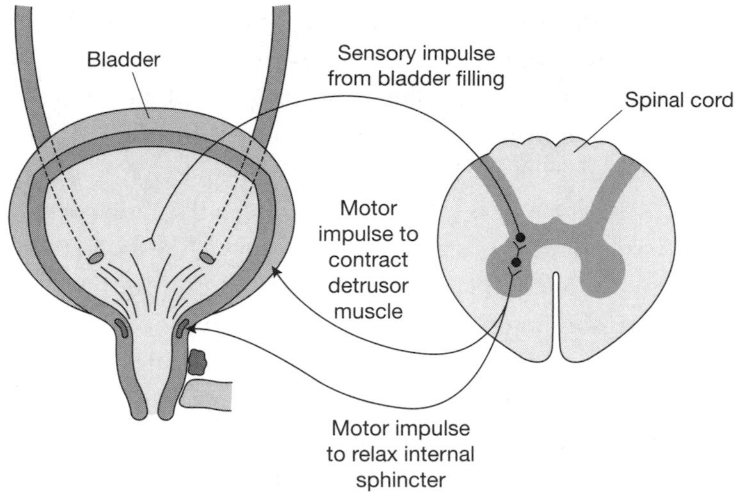

Figure 6.4 The reflex arc for bladder emptying

being consciously expelled. A child's bladder capacity is estimated by age; age in years × 30 plus 30 = ml capacity. Thus, for a six-year-old child bladder capacity would be 210 ml and the child would be expected to visit the toilet around six to seven times a day.

Nervous system maturation is required for bladder control so that the sensory impulses can travel via the spinal cord to the cerebral micturition control centre. Once awareness of the need to void and of the social desirability to control micturition has developed, together with the biological maturation of the nervous system and the social development of the young, this becomes a controlled central nervous system activity which then blocks the reflex arc. Successful control can start at about two years of age when the child can voluntarily relax pelvic floor muscles in order to void.

Bed wetting – nocturnal enuresis

Bed wetting at night is a common experience in early childhood; an alteration of neuromuscular function which is often benign and self-limiting. However, bed wetting can be the cause of much unhappiness in family life. The diagnosis of nocturnal enuresis is made when the involuntary passage of urine, during sleep, occurs in a child aged five years or more, in the absence of any congenital or acquired defects of the nervous system (Kamperis and Djurhuus (2007), cited at www.medicalnewstonight.com) present one of the many reasons for poor control of voiding at night (others include stress, family history, urinary tract infection and developmental delay). They explain how urine output is controlled, in part, by an internal daily clock (circadian rhythm). At night we normally reduce the amount of excreted water, electrolytes and wastes in preparation for sleep. However, some children take longer than others to develop the rhythm; 7 per cent of seven-year-olds wet the bed at night. They suggest that, for some children, it is not the volume of urine produced at night or a bladder that is too small to hold it, but an abnormal kidney circadian rhythm in the way it handles sodium balance in the early hours of the morning.

Mercer (no date, available at www.bedwettingstore.com) shows that wetting the bed at night may be a complex problem. Deep sleep, food sensitivity such as citrus fruits, those who produce more urine than average, those who have small functional bladders (they normally pee more often than their peers), and those who are prone to constipation and thus their bladder expansion is restricted are offered as some of the things to consider when assessing this problem.

Gaining continence

Healthy bladders can be trained by good habits. Drinking adequately flushes out bacteria, but drinking fizzy drinks irritates the bladder. Training girls to clean from front to back avoids them contaminating their lower urinary system with bacteria that normally reside in the rectum, for example e.coli. Children should also be encouraged to void as soon as they feel the urge to micturate, and sexually active girls should void soon after intercourse. Starting school, where toilets are shared and break times fixed, causes problems for some children who will refuse to drink during the day and retain urine until they reach home. Kaushik *et al.* (2007) found that children with free access to toilets consumed significantly more water during the school day.

In assisting parents to help the child gain continence, a thorough assessment of the problem is vital to subsequent support. Questions to ask may include age, principal carer, family attitude to and history of continence, health status and development milestones, recent events in the child's life such as school changes, toilet facilities such as accessibility and the motivation/ability to ask to void, medications and diet/fluid intake patterns. Management will depend on this accurate history taking; some common helpful discussion points can include explanation of continence, reassurance that something can be done, advice on practical organisation such as using waterproof bed covers and having routine times for voiding (in peace!) and twenty-four hour fluid intake management. In all situations the child and the family need to be well motivated to succeed and be praised for effort.

Dehydration and rehydration

Children are susceptible to water loss because of their high percentage of body water and relatively large surface area to mass; dehydration is a leading cause of child suffering worldwide especially where vomiting and diarrhoea are present. A parent/carer and child report is often unreliable; the following observations are important: skin turgor, respiratory pattern, the time blood takes to refill the nail bed, dry mucous membranes, sunken eyes and poor overall appearance (Steiner *et al.* 2004). Friedman *et al.* (2004) also suggest observing for the lack of tear production when assessing young children between one and thirty-six months and palpating for a sunken anterior fontanelle. Loss of excess body water occurs in three ways:

- Isotonic dehydration is when water and electrolytes (especially sodium salt) are lost in equal amounts. The serum sodium remains at 130–150 mEq/litre, normal levels.
- Hypotonic dehydration (hyposmotic) is when the electrolytes are lost and the water concentration rises. The serum sodium is less than 130 mEq/litre.
- Hypertonic dehydration (hyperosmotic) is when there is water loss and retention of electrolytes. The serum sodium will be greater than 150 mEq/litre.

Infants are considered to be mildly dehydrated with 5 per cent water loss, moderately with 10 per cent and severely with 15 per cent. In the dehydrated older child the losses are lower at 3 per cent, 6 per cent and 9 per cent.

Children may be less inclined to eat when dehydrated, be less active and more irritable. Body weight may have been lost but blood pressure may be stable, although the pulse rate will rise as the circulating blood volume reduces. Tissue turgor begins to decrease when the child is 3 to 5 per cent dehydrated; this is best examined on the abdomen and thighs, but the obese child may seem to have a normal skin response, and malnourished children may have loss of turgor through their extreme thinness. A dry mouth can be ascertained by running the finger along the mucus membrane where the cheek and tongue meet; observation of the tongue will show it to be smaller than usual and salivation may be reduced. There is a significant loss from sweat if the body temperature attains 38.3 °C or more or if the ambient temperature rises above 32.2 °C. Dehydration often accompanies a fever as metabolic rate rises, respirations increase and insensible loss occurs from the child's large surface area.

Oral rehydration

The best way to introduce water back into the body is through giving oral fluids. The solution recommended by the WHO contains sodium, potassium, chloride, base, glucose and water. Glucose is the preferred sugar because it facilitates the transport of sodium across the bowel wall. The usual recommendation when used to rehydrate children with diarrhoea is that the child takes this drink (volume calculated to the child's weight) each time there is a bowel action. It is also recommended for vomiting children. Small volumes (5–10 ml) of the solution need to be sipped frequently; a large volume taken quickly into an irritated stomach will stimulate the vomit reflex and further increase fluid loss from the gut. The electrolyte replacement is easily purchased in the UK in crystal form, and it can then be readily reconstituted with either cold or boiled tap water as required. Some of these products are flavoured to make them more palatable; the salt taste can be unpleasant and children will spit it out.

Over-hydration

Small babies cannot tolerate large intakes of free water because their glomerular filtration rate is low and they cannot excrete the diluted urine. Fluid retained in the extracellular spaces will produce water intoxication; the brain tissue is particularly sensitive and the child may have a seizure. As the extracellular sodium dilutes, water moves into the cells and cerebral and pulmonary oedema develops. This condition can occur if babies are fed dilute formula milk, take in excess water from bathing and are given inappropriate glucose solutions for thirst.

Replacement of body electrolytes by diet

When children vomit they lose the acidic gastric juices (hydrogen ions); this causes a metabolic alkalosis in their blood. The kidney attempts to conserve the remaining hydrogen ions from the collecting tubules to correct this disturbance as blood is filtered, and in the process losses to urine of potassium occur. The loss of potassium will make the child feel very shaky and increase the irritability of the heart muscle. If they can eat bananas, dates and raisins – which are high in potassium – these foods can be used more safely than potassium supplements to replace it.

Professional athletes can be seen to use both electrolyte fluids and potassium-rich foods, such as bananas and dried fruits, to compensate for potassium loss. As they lose excessive water by sweating they also lose sodium through the skin; their kidneys then conserve sodium, the same process as conserving hydrogen ions, and expel potassium via the kidney. Both these losses of electrolytes, hydrogen ions and sodium result in potassium loss from the body and the need to replace it by oral intake of particular fluids and diet.

Urine

Children need to void regularly to excrete wastes produced from their body metabolism. The volume and constituents of urine give a good indication of healthy function and are often requested by health practitioners when assessing child health/illness. Understanding the safe collection of samples ensures the correct results are used for the child's ongoing management. It is usual practice for the child's normal carer to be required to help.

The average urine volume for children per day can be calculated in relation to their body size; the bigger the child the more urine they will produce in twenty-four hours. Children vary in size at the same age so a good general rule is 0.5 ml per kg per hour. So if a child is 10 kg, s/he will pass 5 ml per hour, 120 ml per twenty-four hours. For the infant under one year who may weigh from 3–10 kg the urine output would range from 36–120 ml per day – on average 80 ml per day (www.intensivecaring.com).

Collecting urine

Urine samples are often required of small children, and there are many ways to catch them! A 'mid-stream' sample is the best, but difficult to obtain if the child is uncooperative. Older children can be washed with water round the perineal area and then instructed to allow some urine to pass into the toilet before they sample the urine into a sterile pot before completing their voiding. Another way is to attach a collecting plastic bag over the urethral opening, easier in boys than girls, or place a collection pad/cotton ball in the nappy/pants/knickers. The parent/carer can also be requested to catch a clean sample from a toddler who is left without a nappy until they void. This method is time-consuming but less traumatic for some children who are sore.

Observing urine

Routine observation of the child's urine is helpful in detecting change in general health as well as for the laboratory test.

- Smell that is strongly ammoniacal may be the sign of infection; or if the child is taking medication it may reflect that of the oral preparation, for example antibiotics. Some foods also produce a characteristic smell in the urine, for example asparagus.
- Appearance should be straw coloured; if concentrated it will be a dark orange, and if diluted a pale lemon colour. Red urine may reflect the diet of the previous day, for example beetroot. Jaundiced babies will have dark orange/brown urine due to the excretion of bile salts which should be excreted through the gut. Pink deposits from small babies are urates, not blood.
- Children normally void urine five or six times per day depending on their drinking volumes and environment conditions (on hot

days they may pee less frequently). Those who are dehydrated may not void for eighteen to twenty-four hours and still not have a distended bladder. However, some children are embarrassed to void in the presence of strangers or in strange environments; standing them or sitting them in an appropriate position will often get results.

Testing urine

Urine testing is a routine activity by health professionals to measure the base line health of the child. Urine sampling is a useful non invasive test for many body functions.

- Protein in the urine is normal in small amounts. This is due to the expulsion of dead cells that slough off from kidney nephrons, ureters and bladder lining. Levels will rise in the presence of infection as white cells are drawn to inflamed tissue.
- Glucose is not usually present unless the child is anxious, for example from injury or chronic stress, or has eaten a large amount of sugary foods and the blood sugar levels are higher than the usual limits.
- Ketones are commonly found in children's urine where they have not eaten recently, for example in the morning if they have not had breakfast or in the evening after a long day at school. Children who are feverish have a raised metabolic demand (their bodies are working faster), as do children who are very active. Their bodies are breaking down their fat reserves to release energy; their glycogen (carbohydrate energy reserves in the muscles and liver) stores are quickly used up if they do not eat. Release of ketones is the by-product of this fat metabolism.
- The acidity of normal urine is 5.5 – acidic. Small children often have a higher score; their urine is more alkaline due to their diet of milk and milk products. Children who have a high vegetable diet may also have an alkaline result. Urine is acid because the kidney is filtering hydrogen ions out to maintain a blood pH of approximately 7.3.
- The specific gravity (SG) of urine is useful to detect dehydration, together with other observable signs such as small and infrequent volume passed. The specific gravity of water is 1,000, so the

more solutes in the urine the higher the number will be. The child with a urine SG of 1,035 will need more fluid input.

Physiology knowledge in practice

Scenario 1

Ken is four years old and wets the bed at night. What explanation can you give to his mother and what advice could help train him to become dry?

Some pointers:

- Ken is still quite young to be dry at night; he may not have a large enough bladder to hold the urine over night and his nervous system may not be mature enough. There may be a family history of being 'late' with this ability.
- He may have lots of drinks before bed time so his urinary system has lots of work to do as he goes to bed – perhaps he could have more drinks during the day and reduce the volumes in the hour before bed so that he has time to excrete the extra fluid.
- He may have been dry at night but since starting nursery school has been bed wetting again. He may be experiencing a different regime for drinking and voiding now and will settle in to this in a few weeks if he appears happy in his new environment.
- He may have a urine infection; he will need to be taken to a health professional if he appears unwell, off his food, has a tummy ache or his urine smells. He may be passing urine more frequently and complaining that it is sore to pee.
- Mum could be invited to discuss her worries and encouraged to give Ken lots of attention and praise when he is dry and not to make a fuss when he wets the bed but console him. She should avoid fizzy drinks that irritate the child's bladder and perhaps have a reward system that appeals to him. A star chart is commonly used.

Scenario 2

Mary and Millie, twins aged twelve years, enjoy their fish and chips each day with plenty of salt and tomato ketchup on the meal. How does their renal system cope with this excess sodium load in their blood? What happens when they slake their thirst with fizzy pop drinks?

The theory

- Salt (sodium) will increase the solute concentration of the plasma and its osmotic (water) pull, thus water will be drawn from the interstitial spaces (ISS) into the blood. This, in turn, will draw water from the cells.
- The more 'concentrated' blood (high solute load of sodium) will stimulate the osmoreceptors in the hypothalamus. This will detect a rise in osmolality in this extracellular fluid and will initiate a neural circuit that results in the conscious sensation of thirst.
- In the kidney, the rise in anti-diuretic hormone (ADH), stops water loss; secretion from the posterior pituitary, mediated via the osmoreceptors, leads to increased water reabsorption at the nephron distal tubule. Small volumes of water urine will be voided.
- As fluid is replaced orally and ingested via the gut into the blood, it dilutes the sodium which reduces the osmolality in the blood. Water moves back into the ISS and cells and excess of water and sodium are eventually flushed from the body. Urine output increases.
- However, the intake of a very sweet drink raises the blood osmolality again, as did the sodium (salt), and increases rather than decreases dehydration and thirst. Water would be better oral fluid for the twins to have with their favourite salty meal.

Extend your knowledge

Van Hoek *et al.* (2007) investigated the circadian variation of voided volume in normal school-age children and published their findings in the *European Journal of Pediatrics*. They found that the children passed the most amount of urine in twenty-four hours during the morning and the least amount overnight. Can you verify this in your experience with children? How do the children you work with balance their fluid intake and output during their day? Think about the reasons for some of them not having this rhythm and then read the paper and find out what the researchers say.

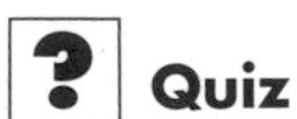

Quiz

1. What are the filtering units of the kidney called?
2. How much water is there in the body of an infant compared to an adult?
3. What do we mean by the 'compartments' of water in the body?
4. Explain water balance in a child compared to an adult.
5. What would be the average daily intake for a child of four years at a weight of 16.2 kg?
6. How many times is the kidney redesigned in foetal life?
7. Why is amniotic fluid vital to foetus development?
8. How much urine will the infant pass in the first ten days of life?
9. What are the basic conditions that are needed for a child to be continent?
10. How does a bladder work?
11. What would the bladder capacity be for a six-year-old child?
12. What is nocturnal eneuresis?
13. What should be considered when assessing a child who wets the bed at night?
14. How would you observe a child for dehydration?
15. What does isotonic dehydration mean?
16. What is the best way to re-hydrate children and justify your answer?
17. Why might a child have a seizure if it is given too much water too quickly after being dehydrated?
18. What foods are good to eat if a child is losing sodium in sweat and its kidneys are excreting potassium?
19. How can you collect a sample of urine from a two-year-old?
20. What might the colour of urine tell you?

Chapter 7

The digestive system

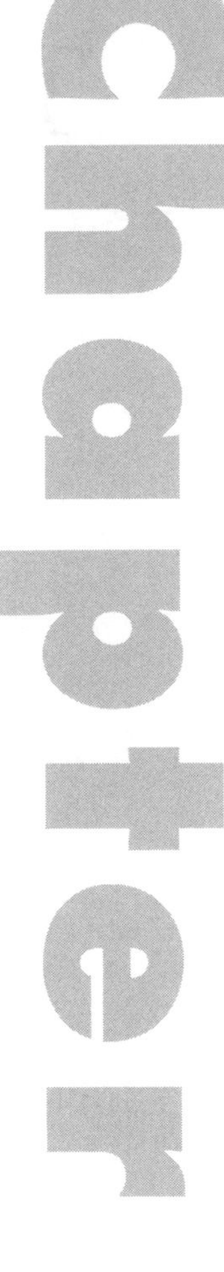

- The developing gut
- The mouth
- Teeth
- Reflexes of the mouth and throat
- The stomach
- The small intestine – duodenum and ileum
- Weaning
- Failure to thrive
- Calorie needs
- The liver and blood glucose balance
- Physiological jaundice
- Bowels
- Stools

THE DIGESTIVE TRACT breaks down ingested food by mechanical and chemical processes, prepares it for absorption and eliminates water and waste products. From the throat to the anus a smooth muscle tube moves food by peristaltic action which is controlled by the autonomic nervous system and action of hormones.

In the mouth, food is broken down by the teeth (a mechanical breakdown) and mixed with a moisturising saliva containing the digestive enzyme (a chemical breakdown) amylase which starts the digestion of carbohydrates such as starch to glucose. The bolus of food moves down the oesophagus into the stomach through the cardiac sphincter, where mechanical breakdown by the three layers of muscles churns the food bolus. In the stomach many substances are secreted into the ingested food; water makes the contents more fluid, mucus protects the stomach lining, hydrochloric acid helps to kill ingested bacteria and activate other digestion processes; the intrinsic factor allows absorption of iron and an enzyme, pepsin (and renin in the infant), commences the chemical digestion of proteins.

The fluid 'chyme' then moves into the duodenum, which is the first part of the small intestine, through the pyloric sphincter. Here, bile, a waste product of the liver, and pancreas enzymes continue the chemical digestion of carbohydrates, fats and proteins. The food then passes into the next sections of the small intestine, the jejunum and ileum. The ileum is where absorption of nutrients tales place; the small capillaries of the blood system transport them into the hepatic portal system and thence to the liver for distribution to the body tissues.

Waste products, such as fibre and excess bile, are then moved through the caecum (a valve) to the large intestine called the colon. Here water is reabsorbed to the blood system together with vitamin K and B complex, which have been manufactured by bacteria living in that part of the gut. The waste is retained in the lower part of this section, the rectum, until stretch receptors initiate defecation (Marieb and Hoehn 2007) (Figure 7.1).

The developing gut

The anatomical combinations that eventually result in the digestive system explain how some infants are born with strange anomalies such as the oesophagus and trachea joined together, abdominal

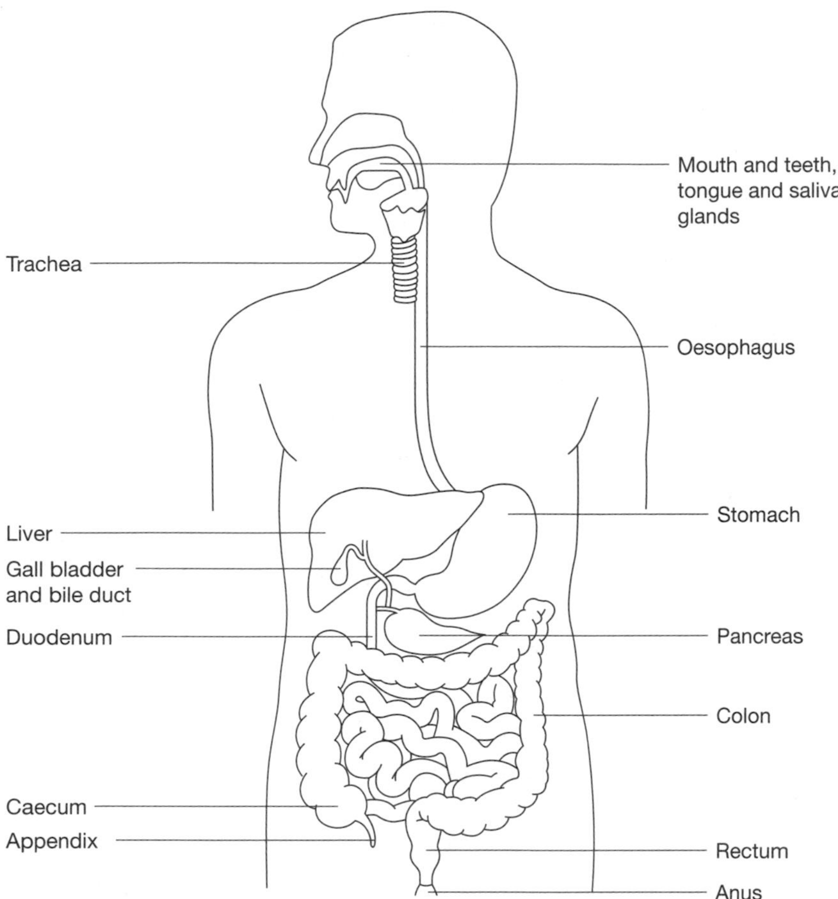

Figure 7.1 Digestive tract

contents which have grown outside the skin covering of the abdomen rather than inside it, and an imperforate anus.

In the embryo, the primitive digestive tract is a tube evolving from three separate parts: the foregut, the midgut and the hindgut which develop separately from the yolk sac. The foregut gives rise to the pharynx, lower respiratory system, oesophagus, stomach, first and second sections of the duodenum, liver, pancreas and biliary apparatus. The midgut gives rise to the duodenum through to the transverse colon. The hindgut develops into the rest of the large intestine to the anus. Due to herniation of the midgut into the umbilical sac at week six to ten of foetal life, the mesentery, which is a skin keeping all the gut in position, is fixed at the top in the left upper quadrant of the abdominal cavity by the ligament of Treitz and at the bottom in the right iliac fossa.

The mouth

The function of the mouth is to take in food and water and prepare them for chemical digestion and absorption as they pass through the gut. Lips, teeth, tongue, hard palate, three pairs of salivary glands and muscles of the face all help in this process; any malformation of the anatomy will make ingestion of food problematic.

When a baby is born it is suddenly separated from its source of nutrients in the maternal circulation; thus the neonate may lose 5 to 10 per cent of its body weight due to this shock at birth. At birth the infant's lips are well adapted to closing round a nipple to feed. They are usually parted at rest and show 'sucking blisters' or *pars villosa*. These keep the seal when the baby sucks. At rest, the back of the mouth is firmly closed with the tongue against the palate if not swallowing. When feeding, the baby draws the nipple far back into the mouth, then squeezes milk by elevating the dorsum of the tongue from the front to the back against the hard palate. The gums then open, the tongue slides forward and the system refills with milk. This stripping and swallowing cycle then repeats (see Figures 7.2 and 7.3). There is usually a rhythm of one breath to one or two swallows. The efficiency of this system increases at birth (from week forty of gestation).

Very premature infants do not have this sucking ability and may have to be fed by tube until they are mature enough, and all young babies with blocked noses will have this rhythm broken and may not feed adequately. Infants appear to accept both breast and bottle nipple

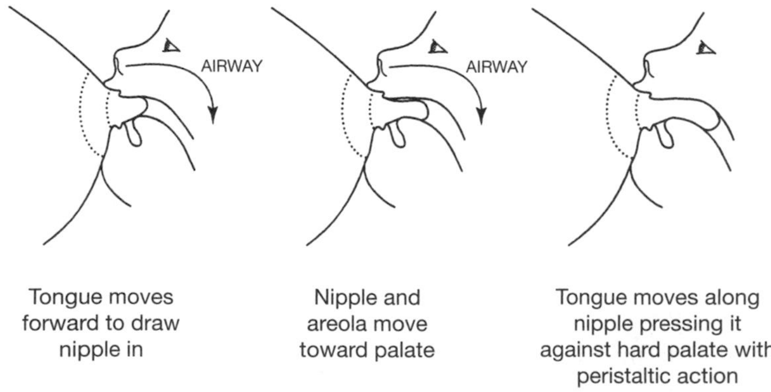
AIRWAY
AIRWAY
Tongue moves forward to draw nipple in
Nipple and areola move toward palate
Tongue moves along nipple pressing it against hard palate with peristaltic action

Figure 7.2 Sucking from the breast

quite readily, but as the skill is perfected nipple preference becomes evident and breastfeeding may become more difficult if the baby is fed complementary or supplementary infant formula milk from a bottle. The teat of the breast and the bottle are different in shape and texture; small babies are expert at the one they prefer. Many mothers have a battle to wean their child off the breast and try many shapes of teat to pacify their offspring. Yet others find that if the bottle is used for a short period of time due to sore nipples or exhaustion from the baby's constant snacking, the baby will not work at the different sucking skill to gain nourishment from the breast, having found it easier to gain food from the artificial source.

The pharyngeal-oesophageal swallow is a primitive function but the child's mouth quickly learns discriminative and motor skills. In the first few months the suck and swallow will progress to manipulation of more solid food without gagging. Only small amounts of saliva containing the enzyme amylase are produced by the salivary glands in the neonate with little enzyme function; however, these develop full function by the age of two. All infants have taste and smell present at birth, and they all can soon learn to enjoy sweet tastes distinguished by the taste buds at the tongue tip, soft palate and inside of the cheek. If oral medications are sweetened children are usually happy to cooperate if a small amount is introduced at the front of the mouth. Breast milk is sweeter than artificial feeds, thus, breastfed infants appear to enjoy fruits as their first foods. The ability to suck semi-solid food, bite and chew, appears at five to six months and lumpy food can be tolerated at six to seven months, a 'sensitive period' for this motor ability. However, many children will gag or spit out lumps for some months over their first year.

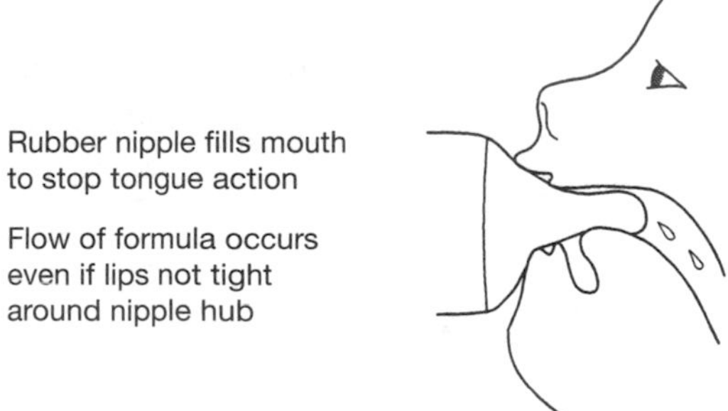

Rubber nipple fills mouth to stop tongue action
Flow of formula occurs even if lips not tight around nipple hub

Figure 7.3 Sucking from the bottle

Teeth

Teeth may be present in the newborn but generally they start to erupt at about six to eight months; the lower two central incisors are usually first. Some infants do not commence teething until twelve months, although they have dribbled and chewed their fists for weeks. Teething leads to an increase in salivation and babies may have loose stools, nappy rash, a raised temperature and cough, but there is controversy on this point. There is also controversy on symptoms experienced by some babies, as some have no problems at this time and others are unhappy for days (www.teething-babies.co.uk). The complete set of deciduous teeth numbers twenty, and is achieved by thirty months; they should be carefully guarded. Fluoride builds strong, decay resistant enamel on the outside of the tooth and reduces caries (tooth decay) by 70 per cent. It has been added to city water supplies for over fifty years, although only 14 per cent of the UK population receives it at present. Toothpaste also contains fluoride and should be used in moderation if local water has been treated as children will usually swallow it. Mottling of the teeth can occur if too much is absorbed but this does not increase problems with caries. Tooth brushing should commence at six months to remove the plaque that deposits there; bacteria change sugars to acids which eat away at the tooth enamel (www.aboutkidshealth.ca). Sugary drinks and lack of tooth brushing were shown to increase the development of caries in eleven to fifteen year olds in a study of 500 UK schoolchildren by Levine *et al.* (2007).

The young child has no molar teeth so cannot chew thoroughly, and the deciduous teeth are blunt. At six to eight years the deciduous teeth will begin to be lost in the same order they were grown, but the full set of adult teeth may not arrive until adolescence. Today there are many adults without the full set of thirty-two teeth which include the 'wisdom' teeth molars. This may be an inherited characteristic such a small mouth or the effect of food eating changes over generations.

Reflexes of the mouth and throat

There are neural reflexes which protect the airway from occlusion; the pharynx is poorly designed to allow the simultaneous passage of food and air. Swallowing is an autonomic reflex for the first three months of life until the striated muscles in the throat establish cerebral connections but by six months the baby is capable of swallowing, holding food in the mouth or spitting it out. Small children need to be supervised at meal times till they are safe with solid foods. Goyal and Mashimo (2006) explain how swallowing is a complex activity and can be described as three phases: preparatory, transfer and transport. The act of swallowing has both voluntary and involuntary components; the transfer of food across the mouth and into the pharynx are the involuntary phases. This swallow activity is coordinated by the brain stem but involves many nerve circuits and types of muscle groups.

The stomach

The stomach normally holds food for four to six hours and has many important functions in digestion; its capacity increases as the child grows.

Prior to birth the gastrointestinal tract is filled with fluid and the remnants of the developing bowel lumen as it grows and sheds the lining. By five months, the foetus is swallowing small amounts of amniotic fluid, dead hair and skin cells and bile excreted from the liver. Together they form the meconium which is eventually passed through the rectum as the infant's first stool and proof of anal function.

At the first few breaths after birth the infant swallows air; after three hours the whole gut contains gas. As the child continues to feed orally, so gas is taken in. A 3.5 kg baby will take in 100 ml of milk feed in fifteen minutes and the same volume of air. The best position to 'burp' an infant is to hold it sitting supported at the back and neck so as to allow the gas to bubble up a straight oesophagus. Patting a baby on the back may be comforting for the carer to have a physical contact, but gas will rise to the top of 'a bag of fluid', so if the stomach is positioned with the cardiac sphincter of the stomach upright the gas will rise up to the mouth. 'Windy' babies are often more comfortable propped up for an hour, carried upright looking over the carer's shoulder, or placed on their abdomen over a carer's lap after a feed, so that wind can be expelled, before being put to sleep flat (supine) on their backs. At present, with the advice to lay infants only on their backs to avoid cot deaths from suffocation, many mothers are reluctant to use the face-down position, even under constant supervision.

The position and shape of the infant stomach is high in the abdomen and is orientated transversely rather than vertically as in the older (seven to ten years) child. The capacity of the stomach changes with age (see Table 7.1). Emptying time for the newborn's stomach is two and a half to three hours (for the five-year-old it is three to six hours). At birth the abdomen and thorax are of equal circumference; as all muscles in the body are poorly developed initially, the abdomen will appear prominent in early childhood. Muscle development also affects the digestive tract and lower oesophagus tone, an important barrier to preventing the reflux of stomach contents. The functional immaturity of the lower oesophagus 'sphincter' (Figure 7.4) also leads to episodes of inappropriate relaxation, and the short intra-abdominal length of this tube contributes to the young child being able to readily bring back their meals.

Hydrochloric acid is present in the stomach at birth but falls too low to facilitate much digestion of protein by the stomach enzyme pepsin or destruction of ingested bacteria. The bottle-fed neonate will be vulnerable to orally transmitted gut infections from poor sterilisation techniques. The pH is nearly neutral (pH 7) due to swallowing of the alkaline amniotic fluid, but, in the first eight hours of life, gastric secretion of acid does commence. The stomach's role at this time is, however, more important for coagulating the casein of milk and controlling its passage to the small intestine. Curd (casein) may stay in the stomach and be gradually broken down over twenty-four hours, whereas the fluid whey will move through to the duodenum within an hour. Acid secretion reaches adult levels at about ten years, when children become less likely to develop gastroenteritis as the acid will kill bacteria from oral intake more completely.

Table 7.1 Stomach capacities by age (ml)

New-born	*1 week*	*2–3 weeks*	*1 month*	*3 months*	*1 year*	*2 years*	*10 years*	*16 years*	*Adult*
10–20	30–90	75–100	90–150	150–200	210–360	500	750–900	1,500	2,000–3,000

The small intestine – duodenum and ileum

Most biochemical and physiological functions are present at birth; secretory cells are functional but mature in efficiency with age. The pancreatic secretions are sufficiently mature for a milk diet, and lactose (milk sugar) can be digested from forty weeks' gestation. This lactase enzyme activity is high in the small intestine at birth, but declines during infancy and is lost by adult life in many individuals. Amylase, a pancreatic enzyme secreted into the duodenum that breaks down carbohydrates, and enterokinase, which is secreted from the ileum mucosa to activate trypsin for the breakdown of protein to peptides, are also present in the neonate gut. In the first three months pancreatic juice contains only a little lipase, which limits the baby's capacity to convert fat into fatty acids and glycerol. Specific long-chain polyunsaturated fatty acids (LCPs) are present in breast milk to feed the large developing brain; thus nature has matched the milk supply to the young human's physiology.

First foods of ground rice and fruits are more easily digested as starch and fructose are simple to digest. It is interesting that in the first six months only small amounts of pancreatic amylase are produced to digest more complex foods. Could it be suggested that this may be a reason for colic at this time? If foods are too difficult to breakdown, the lack of the relevant digestive enzymes allows material to pass undigested to the colon, where the rise in osmotic pressure will draw water from the interstitial spaces and lead to increased peristalsis and loose stools. Cow's milk protein has been identified as a stimulus, both if given to the infant or taken by the breast-feeding mother. However, true colic is self-limiting; infants over six months show a reduction in this condition when a more mixed and solid diet is offered.

Weaning

Weaning programmes are recommended from six months; they incorporate the need to increase the consistency and texture of solid foods at this age (www.babyledweaning.com, www.who.com, www.organix.com). However, some babies are reluctant to try at the first attempt and will gag; they may prefer a smooth texture for a few more weeks. The food will be pushed out of the mouth because they are learning a new method of transferring solids from lips to throat. Saliva, at first, contains little starch digesting enzyme (salivary amylase) but at three months it increases, and cereals can be digested and biscuits sucked soft enough to swallow at six months. Rice is recommended as a first cereal because of the possibility that an allergy to gluten may occur in some children (1:2,000 incidence). Wheat, oats, rye and barley contain gluten but rice and maize do not. Choking on large lumps is still a danger at this age. Fruits with pips, seeds or thick skins, nuts or highly spiced foods need a mature digestive system, good teeth and the ability to avoid accidental inhalation for efficient digestion. After six months a mix of foods is necessary to provide sufficient energy, trace elements (especially iron) and vitamins. Sodium (salt) levels will be excessive if unmodified cow's milk is given as the only milk source; cow's milk protein is also difficult for the child under one year to digest and, if given as the main 'food', is thought to be one of the common causes of iron deficiency anaemia in this age group. Salty foods should be restricted in childhood because sodium intake has been implicated in the onset of hypertension and cardiovascular damage in adulthood. Bags of crisps and other salty snacks are not recommended as a frequent 'filler'; it is better to offer children fruit as snacks. Food that is dense in calories, offered at routine mealtimes, is preferred so that snacking habits during the day are not encouraged, especially in the under fives, who can be capricious eaters.

Failure to thrive

Children who fail to thrive from feeding problems can be classified under 'too little in', 'failure to utilise nutrients' and 'too much out'. Feeding problems cause many parents to seek professional help; it is helpful to reflect on the need to eat. Eating is a physiological response to the body's requirement for energy to function and grow, it is a social activity and it is a habit. If the child does not eat it will die.

Too little food intake can be due to physical feeding difficulties such as cleft palate or sore mouth, excess vomiting which itself can be the symptom of a multitude of conditions, anorexia where the child refuses to eat for psychological reasons, ignorance of feeding requirements such as parents with learning difficulties or poor education and economic poverty where there is just not enough understanding or money to buy and generate healthy meals for the family.

Failure to utilise nutrients includes genetic conditions such as cystic fibrosis where the energy to breathe and the constant chest infections keep the child's body constantly working hard and using energy for this rather than growth, congenital diseases such as gluten allergy where the ileum remains inflamed and unable to absorb nutrients presented to it, or severe infestations such as intestinal worms which latch onto the gut and draw off nutrients from the blood and gut.

Too much out includes infections such as e.coli and campylobacter which inflame the ileum and prevent water absorption so the stools remain dilute, 'toddler diarrhoea' which is common when the child moves from baby diet to a more mixed lumpy diet of adult foods and their digestion processes are immature, and chronic conditions such as diabetes where glucose is voided in the urine if no insulin is available to allow cells to access their energy source from the blood; the glucose pulls water out of the body as it is excreted through the kidney.

Calorie needs

Children need to eat to fuel their high metabolic rate (rate of fuel burning) and to support their energy expenditure for growth. Children's diets are under scrutiny as more UK children become overweight and their behaviour and intellectual performance deteriorates. Baker (2005) reports on the work of Gesch and others who are researching diet and behaviour. The omega 3 and six fatty acids and vitamin E found in diets containing oily fish, show positive results for children's behaviour and school success. Increases in height and changes brought about by development milestones leads to changes in shape and basic metabolic rate; as surface area reduces to body mass and size increases, so calorie needs per kilogram reduce over childhood. BMR, the use of fuel (energy sources) when the individual is at rest, is where energy released from food meets the needs of the heart, lungs, nervous system and kidneys, and excess is lost as heat through the skin. The skin surface area, in square metres, is calculated from the height and weight of the individual. However, age, sex, menstruation, eating/starving, exercise, fever and thyroid function must all be considered when assessing metabolic rate and calorie use for any individual.

The energy required to raise the temperature of 1 kg of water by 1 °C = 1 kilocalorie = 1,000 calories. The UK advice is that women require 1,940 kilocalories per day and men 2,550. Children's requirements are proportional to these values related to their age and other considerations.

The calorie needs of the pre-school child (one to five years), however, are not as high as that of the infant but small children still need frequent and varied meals with snacks consisting of foods high in nutritional value. Cereal and milk products contribute the most to energy, supplying protein, iron, calcium, zinc, vitamin A, vitamin B and riboflavin. Fruit drinks contribute to vitamin C intake. Thus, a good breakfast of cereal with milk, toast and a drink of fruit juice is ideal for children before starting the school day.

For the average child who is growing and developing normally and has a normal activity level counting calories is usually not necessary. In general, though, knowing how many calories a child needs each day can help plan their nutrition and make sure they are eating a healthy diet. Being familiar with calorie requirements can also be helpful in evaluating children with failure to thrive, who are gaining weight well, and for children who are overweight. Currently 8.5 per cent of six-year-olds and 15 per cent of fifteen-year-olds are obese (www.weightlossresources.co.uk). For younger children, calorie recommendations and average energy needs depend on their age (Table 7.2). Remember that these are just averages; some children require more calories and some will require less. The amount of calories that allows a child to grow normally is likely to be what is 'enough' for him.

Table 7.2 Estimated average requirements for dietary energy

Age	*Average calorie needs each day*
0–5 months	650
5–12 months	850
1–3 years	1,300
4–6 years	1,800
7–10 years	2,000

Source: www.keepkidshealthy.com.

Table 7.3 Estimated average requirements for dietary energy

Boys	*Average calorie needs each day*
11–14 years	2,500
15–18 years	3,000

Source: www.keepkidshealthy.com.

Table 7.4 Estimated average requirements for dietary energy

Girls	*Average calorie needs each day*
11–14 years	2,200
15–18 years	2,200

Source: www.keepkidshealthy.com.

In addition to age, for older children, calorie requirements are also determined by their sex, with boys, in general, requiring more calories than girls (see Tables 7.3 and 7.4). Other factors include a child's size, body composition and level of activity. A very active teenager at the top of the growth charts will likely need many more calories than a smaller and/or less active child.

The liver and blood glucose balance

The liver is a large organ that lies in the right hypochondrical and epigastric regions of the abdominal cavity under the diaphragm within the rib cage. It has many vital functions; several of its activities are linked closely to digestion of food. It receives all the circulating blood and filters out substances such as alcohol and drugs. It breaks down worn out red blood cells which it excretes as bile into the duodenum to help digest fats and redirects absorbed nutrients received via the hepatic portal vascular system to all organs and tissues. It stores vitamin A and other fat soluble vitamins and makes plasma proteins. There are three main plasma proteins: globulins which protect the body from infection, albumen which maintains blood viscosity and fibrinogen that is involved in the clotting cascade response to injury.

One important action of the liver is to maintain blood glucose levels so that the brain can continue to function regardless of food ingestion. It does this by responding to two pancreas enzymes. Insulin facilitates glucose entry to body cells in the fed state (including liver stores which take in glucose from the blood and convert it to glycogen and lipid (fat) stores), and glucagon which facilitates liver glycogen stores to be released into the blood as glucose in the starved state (Geissler and Powers 2005).

Quiros-Tejeira (2007), in investigating the liver function of overweight youths, found worrying glucose metabolism abnormalities that would eventually lead to adult pathologies such as heart disease and diabetes if they remained obese. He found that their body cells were becoming resistant to insulin, their blood sugars were remaining consistently above the normal range of 4–7 mmols per litre and glucose stored as glycogen in the liver and muscles was being processed to fat rather than released back to the blood as an energy source for cell function. These fat boys were developing cirrhosis of the liver in the same way that adults were responding to excess consumption of alcohol.

Physiological jaundice

The neonatal liver is functionally immature. It has low levels of the enzyme required for production of bilirubin, formed from the breakdown of the 'haem' of haemoglobin found in the red blood cells. This enzyme system takes the first two weeks after birth to develop to a normal functioning level. Thus, physiological jaundice frequently occurs at this time. Jaundice occurs when there is a rise of bilirubin in the blood. Normal levels are below 1.5 mg/ml and jaundice is detected if the levels rise above 3 mg/ml. It can be seen in the sclera, soft palate and skin of the infant because the bilirubin is retained in the blood plasma and excreted via the kidney rather than excreted by the liver into the gut. Normally the liver will bind bilirubin to albumin in the plasma and add a sugar molecule to form a 'conjugated bilirubin', which is water soluble and excreted in the bile via the gut. If this process does not happen the bilirubin is not 'conjugated' to sugar and is lipid (fat) soluble, which is why it permeates into the adipose (fat storing) body tissues of the infant.

Physiological jaundice, present in 15 per cent of healthy breastfed infants, is caused by this immature hepatic function and a rise in the bilirubin load from red blood cell destruction which rapidly increases within twenty-four hours of birth. This breakdown of red cells occurs more frequently in the neonate because their red cell life span is seventy days as compared to 120 days for adults and their foetal haemoglobin levels are high. Physiological jaundice is made more severe if the infant becomes dehydrated due to inadequate feeding because the lack of circulating fluid allows the concentration of bilirubin to rise and the child becomes sleepy as the brain becomes toxic; the risk of becoming more dehydrated then increases. If enteral feeding, by breast or bottle, is not encouraged, bilirubin will also be reabsorbed back from the gut rather than expelled in the stools; bile in the gut will make the stools dark green and loose because bile is an irritant to the gut lining, increasing the dehydration risk.

Bowels

The large intestine consists of the colon, rectum and anus. It is in the colon that water is reabsorbed to the blood circulation, solid matter is compacted ready for expulsion and 'friendly' (commensal) bacteria manufacture vitamin K and B complex. The rectum is a straight muscular tube with a simple mucus membrane lining that is thick but loosely connected to the muscle coat beneath. Constipation, where solid stools are retained in this section of the large bowel, can stretch and damage this lining which can lead to eventual prolapse. The smooth muscle here is relatively thick compared to the rest of the digestive tract; its function is to expel a solid waste. Waste is retained in the rectum by two sphincter muscles: the internal anal sphincter, at the superior end of the anal canal, and the external sphincter composed of skeletal muscle (Figure 7.5) which lies at the inferior end. The external sphincter is enervated from the fourth sacral vertebra and is normally in contraction because it has no antagonistic muscle. Thus, it keeps the anal orifice closed and can be tightened at will. Any medications administered to children rectally must be introduced gently to overcome this tight control, because children will usually tense with anxiety.

Waste products are moved through the large intestine by a stimulus originating in the stomach, when filled after a meal. This peristaltic contraction moves through the whole gut and commonly is experienced at the rectum fifteen minutes after breakfast is ingested. Distension of the rectal wall by more faeces entering from the colon

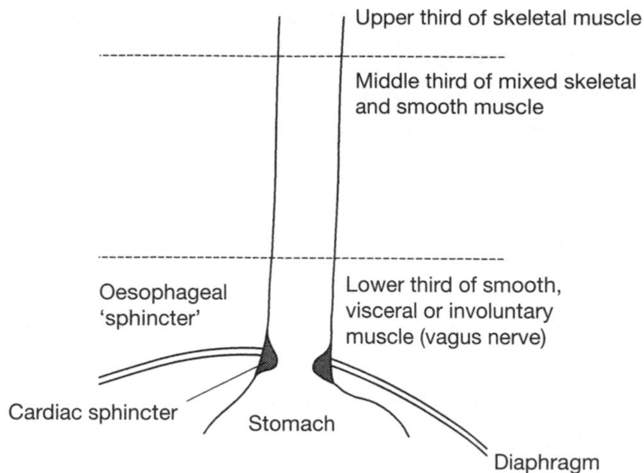

Figure 7.4 The oesophageal sphincter

stimulates the defecation reflex of the internal sphincter. This reflex persists for only a few minutes before it is extinguished. Good training to respond to this reflex regularly will ensure that good bowel habits are formed and comfortable stools passed. If children have to wait to pass a stool they will quickly lose the urge to push, retain the faeces in the colon where water will be extracted and thus a harder, more constipated stool will be formed.

In the infant, a stool is usually passed in relation to eating and the toddler may have a regular 'poo' after breakfast. Some mothers will recognise this fact and 'potty train' their offspring from birth. However, this is a reflex action for more than two years rather than a conscious decision by the very young child. Small children cannot control their bowel until their nervous system has matured to allow them central nervous system control. Their stool is passed simply when the rectum is full.

The external sphincter, under conscious cerebral control, will eventually prevent or allow defecation as appropriate. This is often accompanied by voluntary movements to help expulsion, such as taking a deep breath, closing the larynx and contracting the abdominal muscles. The pressure in the abdominal cavity then rises and forces the faeces out. Again, some mothers recognise this moment and sit the child on the potty successfully and reward the behaviour positively.

This is the start of potty training. However, many children see this as a game and do not understand, while others will resist the

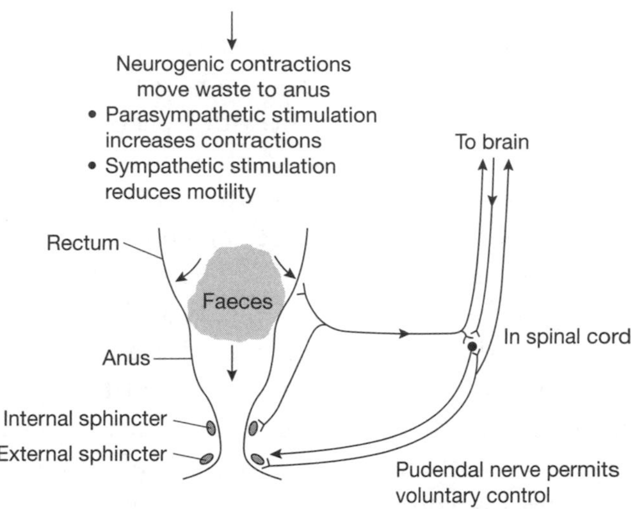

Figure 7.5 Internal and external anal sphincters

urge due to attention-seeking behaviour or anxiety, becoming more and more constipated as the urge fades quickly. At twenty-four to thirty months children may have reached readiness for daytime control of the bowel; they will mimic adult toilet routines, enjoy the attention of having a potty for themselves, understand what is required of them and respond to encouragement and praise (www.babycentre.co.uk). On starting school, where shared toilets may be embarrassing for some children, or where anxiety about punishment is a problem for others, children of five years and above may regress temporarily in this ability. Consistent faecal soiling, however, is abnormal over the age of four years.

Stools

The stools of the newborn (meconium) are odourless, dark green, have a smooth, paste-like appearance and are passed within the first twenty-four hours in about 87 per cent of infants and within 48 hours by 99 per cent. This is not influenced by whether the infant is breast- or bottle-fed (Catto-Smith 2005). After this, the method of feeding will have impact on stool frequency, colour and consistency of the stool. Breastfed babies pass softer, uniformly yellow stools up to five times per day or may, occasionally, pass no stool for up to three days. Bottle-fed babies appear more regular and have fewer bowel actions normally than their breastfed peers. Stool frequency reduces with age with 96 per cent of pre-school children having a normal average range of three motions per day to every other day.

Stools in the first two days of life are composed of digestive juices, desquamated cells and amniotic fluid. The transitional stools are slightly porridge-like; water, casein, fat, fatty acids, mineral salts and live and dead bacteria are present in these faeces. Breastfed babies' stools have a lower pH than babies fed on infant formula milk, due to the fermentative gut flora, b.acidophilus, which produces neutral and acid metabolic waste products. When the pH drops, the faecal enzymes become less active and thus these breastfed babies usually have less nappy rash. Nappy rash occurs when urine and faeces mix; the urea splitting organisms in urine raise the pH and this irritates the infant's delicate skin. Bottle-fed babies have scanty b.acidophilus and pass firmer, paler stools which can smell foul due to fatty curd that is often present with some mucus.

Excess sugar in the diet will act as a mild aperient because sugar increases the osmotic pull of water into the gut and the stools will become more watery. Also sugary drinks will induce tooth decay, provide excess calories and weight gain, or 'fill the child up' between meals so they refuse more nutritious elements of the diet. Toddler diarrhoea, observed as the child moves from the bland to more mixed diet, is usually self limiting but may be the result of too much citrus fruit, coca-cola and chocolate at the expense of fruit and vegetables.

Constipation is usually defined as a stool frequency of less than three times per week, where the child experiences hard painful defecation and may subsequently voluntarily withhold and experience an overflow of faecal fluid. It is common in childhood (3–20 per cent) but more frequent when fibre and fluid intake is restricted (Catto-Smith 2005). School-aged children may not want to visit the school toilets because of embarrassment or restricted access and cow's milk protein allergy has been recently reported as a contributing factor. Increase of fruit and vegetables, high fibre cereals, more exercise and sometimes a short course of laxative medicine are helpful. First choice laxatives for children should be the 'softners', such as lactulose, which pull water into the gut to swell the stool and increase stimulus on the smooth muscle to increase peristalsis. The 'irritant' laxatives may cause the child to have a painful 'tummy ache' if used without discretion.

Physiology knowledge in practice

Scenario 1

Felix is a four-month-old bottle-fed child who is quite chubby. He is a happy baby and very much loved by his grandmother who looks after him during the day for his mother. He suffers colic after feeds. What would you advise his grandmother and mother is the possible reason and what would you suggest they do?

Some pointers:

- *Gut physiology*. Explain how peristalsis works and the size of the stomach in children.
- *Feed requirements – possibly over feeding*. Check Felix's weight and work out his milk feed requirements. A child of four months would be required to have 120–150 ml/kg/24 hours. The amounts change with age. Felix's carers may have been guided by the amounts on the formula tin and ensured he 'finished his bottle' at each meal. Children do not take exact amounts throughout the twenty-four hour period; breastfed babies are better able to control their needs whereas a bottle-fed baby will have feeds presented to them. Check if he is regurgitating feed, which he will if his stomach is too full, or takes a long time to complete his bottle – spending time sucking the teat for comfort rather than nourishment.
- *Winding a child*. This is important to allow the air that is taken in while sucking to come to the top of the stomach and flow up through the oesophagus. Explain how one can sit a small baby up in a seat after feeds to allow this to happen gently rather than expect it to happen immediately. Wind trapped in the gut gives pain as it stretches the lumen of the tube. In the evening Felix may have air trapped in his gut from all his day feeds.
- *Routines*. These are important with children and should start from birth. If Felix begins to understand when he is fed, played with, expected to be in his cot/pram with his toys he will reduce

his demanding of attention which, perhaps, has led his carers interpreting his cries as hunger.

Scenario 2

Sophie, aged eight years, has holes in her back teeth. Her dentist advises her mother that they will soon be replaced but to encourage her to brush her teeth regularly and to avoid sweet, sugary drinks. Explain the physiology behind this conversation and the need for Sophie to gain good teeth cleaning habits.

The theory

- *Structure of the teeth.* Teeth lie in the sockets of the mandible and maxilla. They have different shapes: incisors, canines, pre-molars and molars. All have the same structure of a crown above the gum covered with enamel made of calcium over the dentin and pulp cavity. The root lies beneath the gum and is connected to the crown by the 'neck'.
- *Eight-year-old dentition.* Primary dentition of deciduous teeth which appear at six months and complete at two years – twenty teeth. At six to twelve years they fall out as the roots are absorbed and adult teeth erupt. The adolescent has all permanent teeth and at seventeen to twenty-five should have thirty-two. Often wisdom teeth, the back molars, do not erupt in an anatomically small mouth.
- *Plaque.* Plaque occurs where sugar and bacteria stay on the enamel surface. Bacteria acids dissolve the calcium in the enamel and the organic matrix the calcium is held in is then digested by protein digesting enzymes. Brushing teeth regularly cleans this plaque off the teeth surface. If plaque is left on the teeth it becomes 'chronic'. This is where the plaque calcifies to a calculus called tartar. This disrupts the seal between the teeth and the gum and it becomes infected. This is called gingivitis. This inflamed area is invaded by white blood cells called lymphocytes and they collect in pockets round the tooth and dissolve the bone. This will allow the teeth to become loose and fall out.
- *Tooth brushing technique.* Teeth should be brushed from the gum to the tooth surface as this takes plaque away from the gum. They should be brushed on the inside and outside surfaces with a soft brush that is regularly exchanged and toothpaste that

contains fluoride. Teeth should not be 'scrubbed' with a side to side motion as this will wear the enamel away and allow bacteria entrance to the sensitive dentin where infection will occur. The mouth should be washed out with clean water and the residues from tooth brushing spat out and not swallowed because fluoride will be absorbed in the gut and may overdose the child who lives in a fluoridated water zone.

Extend your knowledge

Cole *et al.* investigated the phenomenon of thinness in adolescence in their 2007 survey 'Body mass index cut offs to define twinness in children and adolescents'. Read the paper and think about the variables one would have to consider in assessing thin teenagers.

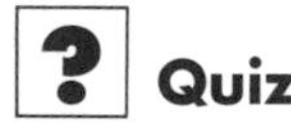

Quiz

Use the word search to find the answers.

C	H	E	M	I	C	A	L	C	F	G	G
E	S	R	R	A	C	I	D	L	L	Y	H
M	M	O	U	T	H	G	L	M	C	S	Z
E	O	E	E	A	T	U	T	E	E	T	H
C	O	A	Y	S	O	C	I	K	U	K	J
H	T	S	D	U	O	D	E	N	U	M	U
A	H	F	G	L	P	J	K	V	X	W	S
N	P	A	O	I	U	F	H	L	N	Y	W
I	N	N	H	S	T	O	M	A	C	H	K
C	X	U	B	N	N	P	U	I	G	A	E
A	H	S	O	L	A	C	A	E	C	U	M
L	P	E	R	I	S	T	A	L	S	I	S

1 Chews food to form bolus.

2 Cuts food up to small pieces ready to swallow.

3 Tube from mouth to stomach.

4 Four- to six-hour reservoir in the gut for ingested food.
5 Where the pancreas enzymes act.
6 Where nutrients are absorbed.
7 Valve between the small and large intestine.
8 Where vitamin K is made.
9 Where solid excreta is expelled from the body.
10 Type of muscle that forms the gut tube.
11 pH of the stomach.
12 Rhythmic movement of the gut when food is ingested.
13 Type of digestion that changes proteins to amino acids.
14 Type of digestion that breaks food ingested down to smaller pieces.

Chapter 8

The reproductive system

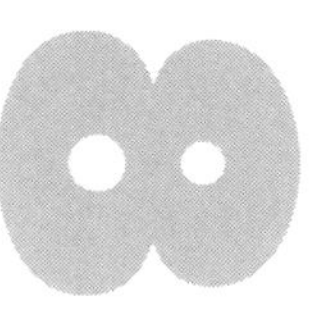

- Male or female – the embryology
- Changes after birth
- Body composition of lean and fat tissues – sex differences
- Changes in the reproductive system at puberty
- Genetics
- The ovary and ovary cycle
- Menstrual cycle
- Sexually transmitted diseases

ALL LIVING THINGS reproduce, it is the process by which organisms make more organisms like themselves (www.kidshealth.org accessed August 2007), but the reproduction system is not vital for physical survival. The most fundamental and obvious difference between boys and girls lies in the anatomy and physiology of their reproductive systems (see Figures 8.1 and 8.2; see also www.thechildrenshospital.org). Once the exact nature and the extent of the biological sex differences are understood, the environmental influences and experiences which shape the way individual children live and the limitations that they put upon themselves can also be considered. Most small children by the age of three years will have noticed the differences between themselves and naked others, especially if they have bathed together. Many have special names for their 'different bits'. Throughout childhood sex differences are evident, but the most striking changes are those occurring during puberty. It is then that development of the secondary sexual differences are seen in the many changes occurring in body tissues as the reproductive system matures.

Male or female – the embryology

The final 'maleness' or 'femaleness' relates to the genetic sex which is given at conception by the sex chromosome combination, the

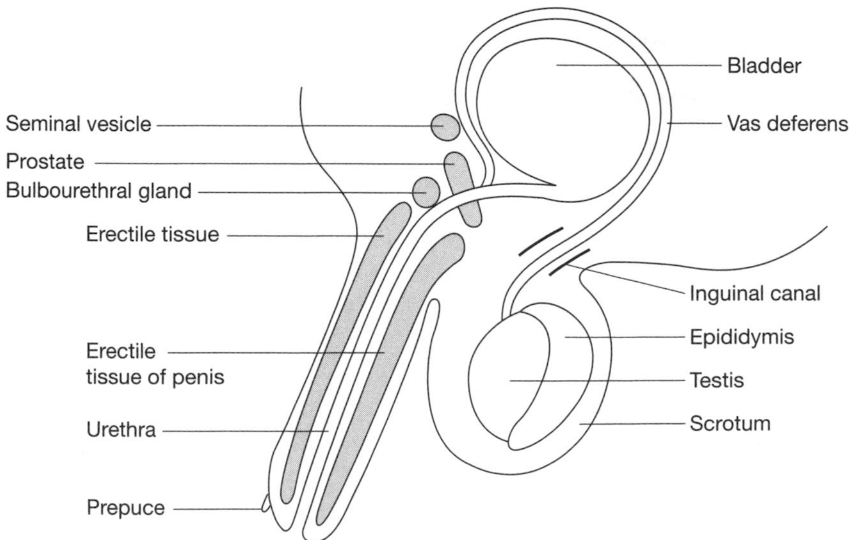

Figure 8.1 Male anatomy

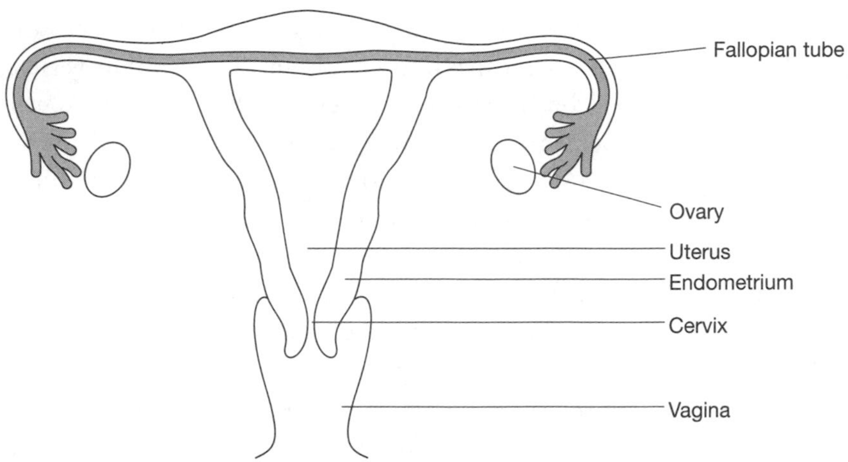

Figure 8.2 Female anatomy

gonad sex which is whether ova (eggs) or sperms are produced, and genital sex which is the outward appearance of the sexual organs. The reproduction system originates in the same tissue for both sexes and develops as female until the male sex chromosome influences further changes. There is much room for a range of outcomes.

In the first five weeks of gestation, the foetus has an 'indifferent gonad' made up of two layers, an outer cortex and an inner medulla. After this time, if male, the medulla forms a testis (gonad sex), while the cortex disappears under the influence of the testis-determining factor on the Y chromosome (genetic sex). If no Y chromosome is present, the cortex will develop and the embryo will continue to develop as a female (Marieb and Hoehn 2007).

In the male, Sertoli cells in the testis cause Leydig cells to differentiate and produce androgens which then masculinise the embryonic genital organs (genital sex). As the pre-Sertoli cells start to differentiate they secrete anti-Müllerian hormone which causes the Müllerian ducts (Figure 8.3), the embryonic female tract, to regress. The effect of the Y chromosome, it is thought, starts earlier, at conception, in order to speed up the growth of the male embryo and allow this differentiation before the oestrogen levels of the mother rise and oppose its effect. By the ninth or tenth week the Leydig endocrine cells secrete testosterone, regulated by the chorionic gonadotropin secreted by the placenta. At eight to twelve weeks testosterone will have stimulated growth of the male Wolffian system

(Figure 8.3), the epididymis, vas deferens and the three accessory glands of the prostate, bulbourethral glands and the seminal vesicle, which are completed by fifteen weeks (refer to Figure 8.1). At this time the levels of foetal testosterone are at their highest and testosterone production is boosted by the foetus's own pituitary gland.

If no Y chromosome has influenced development, then by the third month of gestation the female Müllerian system is fully developed. Fallopian tubes and their associated fimbriae, uterus and inner section of the vagina are complete (refer to Figure 8.2).

Germ cell development (development of the sperms and eggs) shows different time scales. In the male, the primordial cells that will produce sperm remain dormant from the seventh week of embryonic development until puberty. In the female, under the influence of two X chromosomes, the primordial germ cells undergo a few more *mitotic* divisions (see Figure 8.3) after this time to develop eggs, and begin *meiotic* division by the fifth month of foetal life (see Figure 8.4). They, then, also remain dormant until puberty.

Circulating sex hormones may also affect the developing nervous system and subsequent behaviour; androgen levels appear to have an effect on the developing brain and eventual 'male behaviour'. Eventual sexual behaviour, sexual orientation and different anatomy may all be related to the embryo's exposure to fluctuating sex hormones from its own development and that of its mother through the placenta

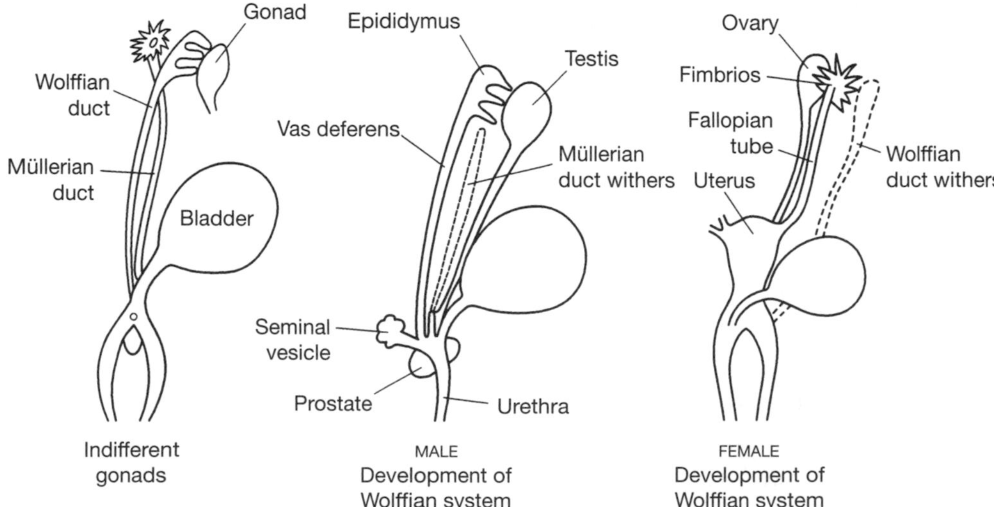

Figure 8.3 The Müllerian and Wolffian systems

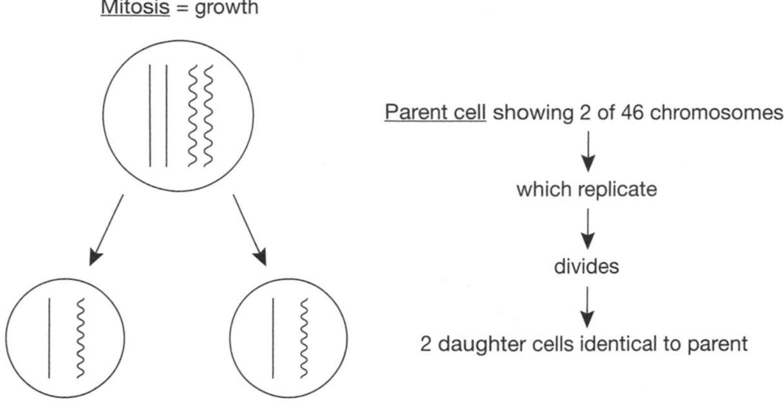
Mitosis = growth
Parent cell showing 2 of 46 chromosomes
which replicate
divides
2 daughter cells identical to parent

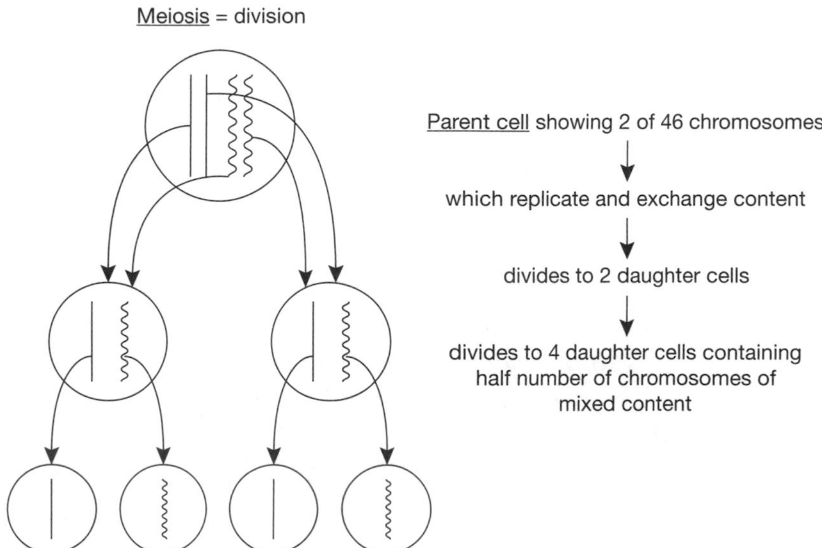
Meiosis = division
Parent cell showing 2 of 46 chromosomes
which replicate and exchange content
divides to 2 daughter cells
divides to 4 daughter cells containing half number of chromosomes of mixed content

Figure 8.4 Mitosis and meiosis

barrier. These effects can be seen in childhood, where boys are generally seen to be more physically aggressive than girls and later in the adult, where sexual orientation may be the result of brain structure determined before birth. Research continues on the nature–nurture debate and the effect of stress hormones on the unborn child. Present views are that chronic stress (raised cortisone levels – see Chapter 9 on the immune system) normally hurts the mother not the baby and that behavioural changes occur after birth when the individual child is exposed to their unique environment (www.news.bbc.co.uk and www.alspac.bristol.ac.uk).

Changes after birth

In the male, testicles usually descend through the inguinal canal to the scrotum, continuing their descent which began one month before birth. They complete their journey as the abdominal viscera grow and testosterone action increases. This descent is necessary for the later maturation of the sperm, which needs a cooler temperature (35–36 °C) than body heat (37 °C). If the testicles are retained in the warmer abdominal cavity, the individual may become sterile as no sperm will develop and the tubules for sperm storage and maturation will become fibrous. However, secondary sexual characteristics will occur because the Leydig cells, which produce the hormone testosterone directly into the blood stream, may still function. Some very premature male infants arrive with undescended testicles as descent is normally at about thirty-eight to forty weeks' gestation: these infants will have to be monitored and minor surgery offered as appropriate. The undescended testes may also be impalpable, abnormal or ectopic where they have followed the wrong route for their descent. Other anatomical aberrations result in hydroceles (fluid sacs) and hernias (protrusions in groin) where there is a persistent *process vaginalis*: the pouch of peritoneum that accompanies the descent of the testes (McCance and Heuther 2006). The seminiferous tubules (sperm transporting tubes) are solid at birth and will not enlarge and open until the testicles enlarge at puberty. The adult testicle weight is forty times that of the newborn baby. The prostate gland and the rectum are the only two major organs in the pelvis at birth. The prostate grows slowly until puberty, then doubles in size over a short period, and then continues to grow slowly for some years. The penis is relatively large in the new baby, and the prepuce imperfectly separated from the glans. The spongy tissue (the erectile tissue that fills with blood when extended) grows in volume throughout childhood (see Figure 8.1). Small male babies can have an erection when their nappy is changed.

In the female, the ovaries are small at birth but large compared to the testicles. They lie in the abdominal cavity in the female infant and only enter the more lateral adult position at approximately six years of age when the bladder descends into the pelvis. A full complement of 400,000 eggs is present at birth in the ovary, which then declines in number over childhood and adult life until menopause (approximately age fifty years). Abdominal injury, infection and drug therapy in childhood can destroy and/or damage this finite supply. The ovarian tissue which encloses the eggs (ova) will grow to twenty times its weight until puberty, when egg maturation and release is stimulated by the hypothalamus. The uterus is large at birth, due to influence of the maternal oestrogen hormone circulated through the placenta, and the size of the cervix is larger than the organ (see Figure 8.2). It lies in the same plane as the vagina until the bladder descends at six years, when it will bend forward in the adult position of anteversian and anteflexion.

In both sexes the breasts may be enlarged in the period immediately after birth, and may discharge clear fluid. This is due to stimulation from the maternal hormone oestrogen: an effect that subsides in the first few weeks of extra-uterine life.

Body composition of lean and fat tissues – sex differences

Under the influence of testosterone, males develop a higher body density than females at all ages and normally show a lower percentage of fat. 'Weight', therefore, must consider the combination of bone, muscle mass and fat deposit. These differences emerge at three to four years and are maintained throughout childhood.

Lean body mass, which includes the essential lipid-rich stores in the bone marrow, brain, spinal cord and internal organs, increases from 25 kg at ten years to 42 kg at sixteen and muscle mass increases from about 12 kg at nine years to 23 kg at fifteen. Girls attain two-thirds, on average, of this lean body mass compared to boys over this time, depending on their genetic inheritance and activity levels. Bunc and Dlouha (2000), in their study to estimate lean mass differences in boys and girls over childhood, show how both boys and girls lose fat to lean mass development as they age and that boys are consistently leaner than girls. Their results:

- boys under the age of ten years have 14.4 per cent fat compared to 25.7 per cent for girls;
- boys aged ten to fifteen years have 13.9 per cent compared to 20.8 per cent for girls.

In all young children the subcutaneous fat overlying the limbs is greater than over the trunk. In puberty, boys lose this limb fat but gain trunk fat. In girls, this change is less marked and fat accumulates specifically round the shoulders, hips and buttocks. The girls have higher amounts of essential body fat because of the tissue laid down in the breast and other sex-specific tissues. The absolute level of storage fat equals that of boys, but because the girl is usually lighter than the boy the relative storage fat is greater. The girl at the end of puberty will have 8–10 per cent more body fat than the boy: her sex specific fat will be about 5 per cent of her total. However, physical activity and socio-cultural influences will produce the larger differences between both males and females.

The fat of the body is contained in a specific connective tissue called adipose tissue. Fat is an energy store, but not all the stores are equally accessible: subcutaneous stores (those under the skin) are used before those round the kidney, for example. Fat appears in the subcutaneous tissues about the sixth month of gestation and is important in temperature control of the newborn: it accounts for 25 per cent of the total weight of the infant. Pads of fat may also be seen on the soles of the feet and in the cheeks of the very young child. Fat cell numbers treble in the first year of life and then increase gradually up to the age of ten years. After this time, there is a gradual increase of size and number to adult levels throughout puberty as circumstances dictate, such as eating excess calories that need to be stored. Some critical periods of adipose tissue development are in pregnancy, childhood and puberty. Genetic and social/economic factors, however, would still need to be considered in the final equation.

Changes in the reproductive system at puberty

Secondary sexual characteristics in male and female

Puberty is a period of sexual maturation, whereas adolescence is a term that includes physical sexual changes but incorporates all the other social and emotional challenges for the young person moving to adult status, depending on their individual cultural expectations. Sexual changes usually commence with a growth spurt, which in boys can begin at ten years or as late as sixteen as timing is influenced by genetic inheritance. The same process occurs in girls but commences approximately two years earlier. Sequence and timing is individual but 50 per cent of children complete the changes in three years. A critical weight has been suggested of 47 kg for girls in the UK to change metabolic rate and trigger hormonal changes, but different race groups may have different critical weights for puberty changes. A simple blood test could identify the beginning of puberty. Research by Wang *et al.* (2004) suggests that leptin, an amino acid made in adipose tissue as it stores glucose, reduces body weight, increases heat promotion and stimulates the hypothalamic–pituitary–gonad axis maturation in puberty. They found that changes in secondary sexual characteristics, such as breast budding (thelarche) and testicle/penis growth, were positively correlated to rising lectin blood levels and BMI measurements for both sexes from nine to eleven years. Thereafter, they found that leptin levels continued to rise in girls but decreased in boys: fat increases in girls in response to oestrogen production and decreases in boys as muscle mass builds.

The sex hormones, testosterone produced in the male testis and oestrogen in the female ovary, are stimulated within a cascade system called the hypothalamic–pituitary–gonad axis (see Figure 8.5, testes, and Figure 8.6, ovary). These hormones combine with others, such as thyroxine and cortisol, to activate the growth of bone and muscle (Marieb and Hoehn 2007). A common hypothalamus gonad-releasing hormone (GnRH) stimulus to the pituitary gland results in the production of follicle stimulating hormone (FSH) and luteinising hormone (LH) which have different effects on the testis and ovary. In the male, LH stimulates the Leydig cells which produce testosterone. Androgens from the adrenal cortex in both sexes stimulate the growth of axilla and pubic hair, skeletal growth, libido, and changes in sweat and sebaceous glands, which give so many teenagers, both boys and girls, personal problems such a distinct body odour and acne. In the ovary, FSH stimulates the maturation of the ovum (in the male the production of sperm in the testes). In the ovary, LH stimulates the theca cells (specialise cells in the ovarian tissue) to produce androgens that are aromatised to oestrogen. LH also facilitates cholesterol movement from the blood to the mitochondria of these cells to be converted to progesterone.

Secondary sexual characteristics are outward signs of changes to adult reproduction function. The specific change seen in boys starts with growth of the testes and scrotum. The growth of the penis and appearance of facial hair occur at the time of increasing body size,

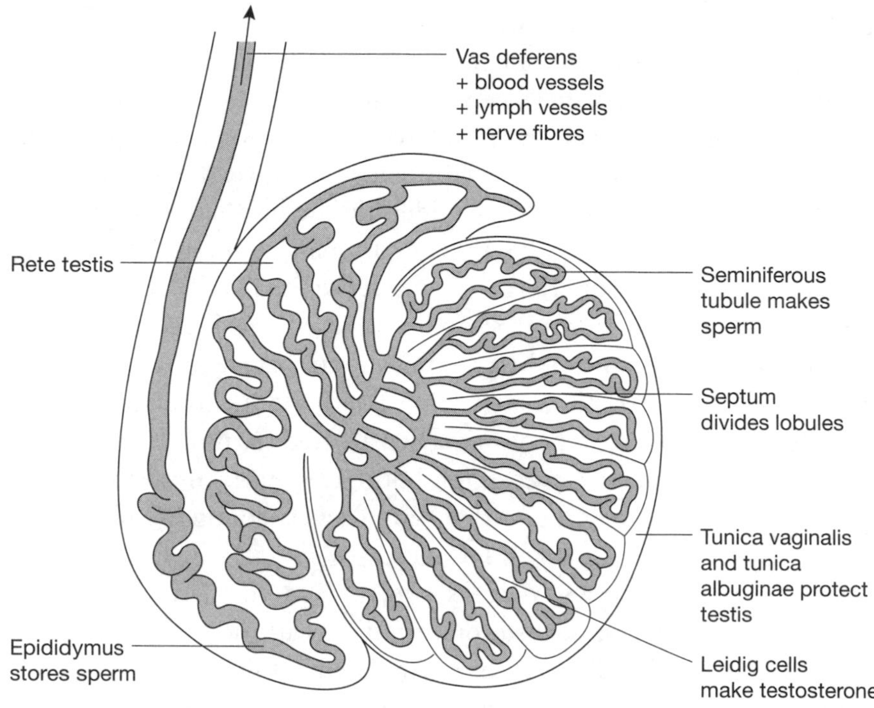
Vas deferens
+ blood vessels
+ lymph vessels
+ nerve fibres
Rete testis
Seminiferous tubule makes sperm
Septum divides lobules
Tunica vaginalis and tunica albuginae protect testis
Epididymus stores sperm
Leidig cells make testosterone

Figure 8.5 Testis

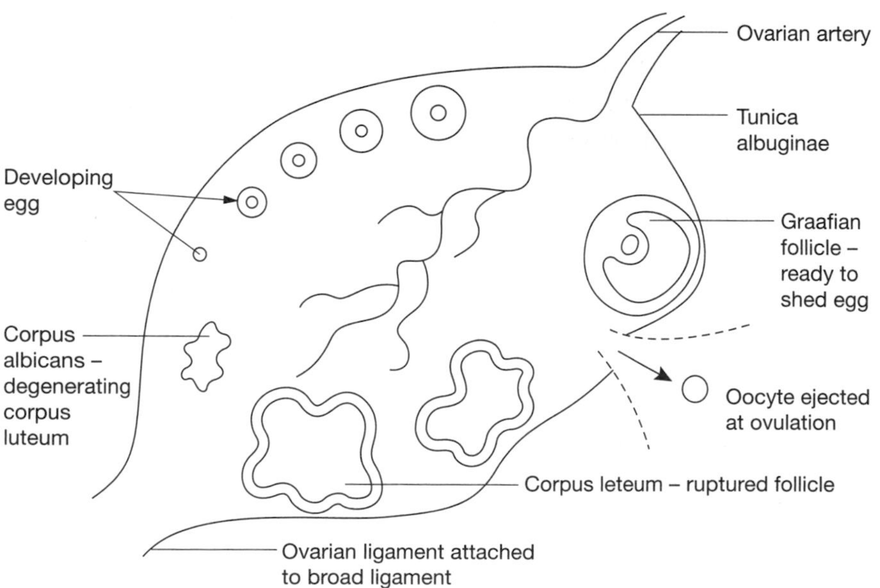
Ovarian artery
Tunica albuginae
Developing egg
Graafian follicle – ready to shed egg
Corpus albicans – degenerating corpus luteum
Oocyte ejected at ovulation
Corpus leteum – ruptured follicle
Ovarian ligament attached to broad ligament

Figure 8.6 Ovary

especially of the skeleton and muscles. The voice then 'breaks' as vocal cords enlarge in the expanding larynx and seminal discharge occurs ('wet dreams') as the seminal vesicles cannulise. The specific changes in girls show enlargement of the breasts, vagina and uterus. Menarche occurs later as growth in height occurs and the pelvic girdle widens.

Genetics

The reason for a mature reproductive system is to ensure survival of the species. Within the developing gonads (testes and ovaries), the sperms and eggs (ova) are prepared for conception and the production of a new individual that has takes on some of the characteristics of both parents. Each cell in the body, other than the sperms and the eggs, has twenty-three pairs of chromosomes which carry all the information needed for the whole body. At any one time, each cell will use only a small part of that information to function. These chromosomes are made up of genes which are small packets of DNA (deoxyribonucleic acid). DNA is made of nucleotides that are combinations of a phosphoric acid, sugar and one of four bases. The sequence of these nucleotides, arranged in threes, is vital as it determines all hereditary traits.

During growth, the chromosomes replicate so that the resulting daughter cells have the exact copy of DNA as their parent cell. This process is called mitosis (see Figure 8.4). In the testes and ova, however, the cells of the gonad undergo meiosis (see Figure 8.4), a halving division, in order to present twenty-three chromosomes, each for conception and the production of a new twenty-three pair (forty-six chromosomes) configuration. In the testes, sperms are produced which contain *either* the X *or* the Y sex chromosome. When combined with the X or X contributed from the female, the male can be seen to contribute to both female or male child as the resulting combinations will show XY or XX (see Figure 8.7).

Genes can be expressed differently depending on the pairing at conception, for example, hair colour. If one gene for blonde hair is matched with its partner for hair that is black, the dominant black gene will block the expression of the recessive blonde gene and the result, the phenotype (what you see), will be black (or dark) hair. However, the blonde genetic inheritance is not lost: the individual

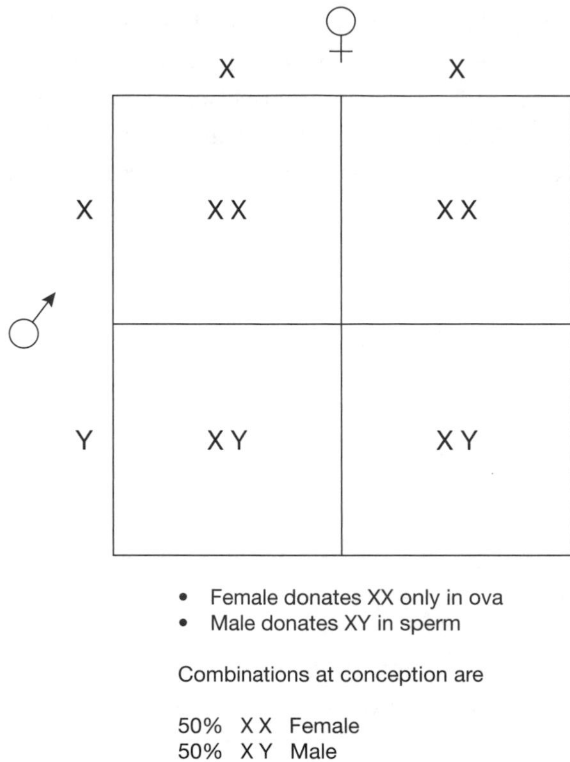

Figure 8.7 Sex inheritance

will carry the blonde gene (the genotype will be a pair that is black and blonde for hair colour) which may reappear at a further conception if the next generation pairing is with a blonde gene. This individual is called heterozygous as s/he carries a pair of choices for hair colour, s/he 'carries' the hidden blonde gene (see Figure 8.8 for possible outcomes in dominance and recessive inheritance). This phenomenon explains the 'carrying' of recessive inherited conditions such as cystic fibrosis. Whereas, the sex inheritance (Figure 8.7) explains the way sex linked conditions, such as haemophilia, are passed from generation to generation. Some traits are produced by co-dominance: this is when one gene does not block the other's expression, such as skin colour, and an intermediate skin colour is seen that reflects the skin colour of both parents. New traits are produced by mutations, when the gene can be deleted or gene material inserted – usually by environmental influences. These new traits can be beneficial or harmful: a beneficial trait might give some advantage over others in the species whereas a harmful trait may make the individual susceptible to disease.

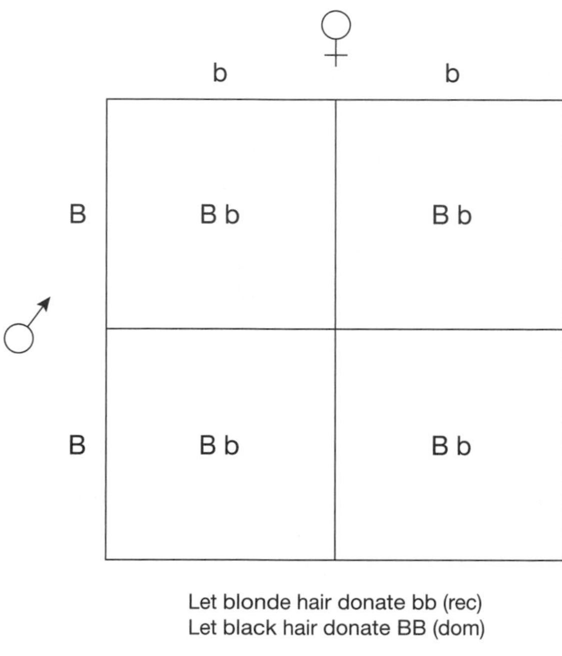

Let blonde hair donate bb (rec)
Let black hair donate BB (dom)

1st generation 100% Bb genotype
– no blonde haired children

* 2nd generation of Bb parents
- 25% black hair (BB genotype)
- 25% blonde hair (bb genotype)
- 50% as parents (Bb genotype)

Figure 8.8 Dominant/recessive inheritance

The ovary and ovary cycle

The two ovaries are the size of a walnut and lie in the lower abdomen attached to a broad ligament either side of the uterus. They each release 'eggs' or ova to the uterus on alternate months via small Fallopian tubes. If one ovary is damaged there is still possibility of ovulation because the second ovary will take over its function. They are present at birth and hold all the 'eggs' for the life of the female.

The ovary has two parts: the germ cell enclosures or follicles, and the surrounding endocrine cells that secrete steroid hormones as well as inhibin, activin, follistatin, anti-Müllerian hormone and oocyte inhibitor (see Figure 8.6). It acts locally to stimulate ova development, and peripherally to: stimulate development and function of the secondary sexual organs; regulate gonadotropin releasing hormone (GnRH) from the hypothalamus; regulate sex-specific physiological function; and support the embryo in early pregnancy.

There are two types of endocrine cells in the ovaries that synthesise hormones from blood cholesterol: the granulosa cells which surround the germ cells and produce oestrogen and the theca cells in the ovary stroma which secrete progesterone. Both these cells, when transformed to luteal cells in the second half of the cycle when no conception has occurred, will produce progesterone. Follicle stimulating hormone (FSH) from the anterior pituitary gland stimulates the granulosa cells to secrete oestrogen, raise the number of luteinising hormone (LH) receptors and secrete inhibin. LH, also from the pituitary gland, stimulates the theca cells to secrete androgens and cholesterol to the mitochondria and their subsequent conversion to progesterone.

Germ cells in the foetal gonads continue to multiply (mitose) to seven million in number, until twenty-four weeks' gestation. After birth, from eight weeks to six months, meiosis (halving of their chromosome number) occurs, and then these cells remain suspended in development until puberty when only 400,000 remain. Hormones from both the granulosa cells round the ovum and the theca cells in the stroma modulate ovum development and secrete directly into the blood to stimulate the secondary sexual characteristics, as GnRH levels from the maturing hypothalamus in the brain rise.

The ovary cycle displays three phases: the follicular, ranging from nine to twenty-three days; the ovulatory, lasting one to three days; and the luteal, lasting thirteen to fourteen days.

- The follicular phase begins just after the levels of FSH and LH begin to rise from their lowest level. This is twenty-four hours before the bleed. FSH starts to rise and continues to rise for the first half of this phase. In the second half of the phase LH starts to rise, LH eventually reaching double the FSH levels. At the same time oestrogen levels rise gradually as the granulosa cells from the dominant follicle move into production (this eventually triggers the negative feedback system to decrease FSH production in the luteal phase). Meanwhile, androgens increase, produced from the theca cells, which leak into the granulosa cells and are aromatised to oestrogen.
- In the ovulatory phase, the LH secretion spikes, together with a smaller one of FSH. The progesterone levels rise and the ovum

is expelled into the Fallopian tube because the LH stimulates an inflammatory response which allows the follicle to rupture. Meiosis (the second chromosome division) occurs in the ovum and the second polar body is formed. The ovum is ready for conception.

- The luteal phase then occurs. Negative feedback from the corpus luteum causes FSH and LH to decline. GnRH pulses are reduced and the progesterone levels increase tenfold. Oestrogen is secreted by the corpus luteum and, if no pregnancy occurs, the oestrogen and progesterone dramatically decline and the bleed starts.

Menstrual cycle

Positive feedback of oestrogen levels on GnRH release in the hypothalamus is the last maturation effect, thus ovulation is not usual in the first menstrual cycles. These cycles are also often irregular because the bleeding is caused by oestrogen levels falling as the Graafian follicles die before they release their ovum.

The menstrual cycle, which can be of any length from nineteen to thirty-six days, is controlled by a group of steroid hormones known collectively as the oestrogens and progesterones. It will occur two years after the commencement of secondary sexual changes, and when body mass, critical adipose mass and skeletal maturation are favourable. It is dependent on LH levels and is usual between the ages of eleven and fifteen years. Height increase stops one to two years after menses start as higher blood oestrogen levels close the epiphyseal plates (growing areas at the end of the bones – see Chapter 2 on the skeletal system).

The menstrual cycle is a local rhythm of the ovary and can be disrupted by situations that affect the ovary function and the function of the pituitary that stimulates and inhibits it. Calorie deprivation, habitual strenuous exercise, stress and depression have all been linked to changes in menstrual cycle function. Oestrogen and progesterone are released from the ovary over approximately forty years of the female fertile period: from menarche to menopause. These hormones are, in turn, controlled by hormones released from the anterior pituitary, FSH and LH. The pituitary hormones themselves are controlled by the hypothalamus hormone GnRH as FSH, LH, oestrogen and progesterone hormones, circulating in the blood throughout the monthly cycle, change. The hypothalamus, also, can be mediated by many other hormones released into the blood. Thus, this hypothalamic–pituitary–gonad axis can be complex even in its normal function.

The uterus lining shows two phases that keep it regularly prepared for conception: the proliferative phase and the secretory phase (see Figure 8.9, uterine lining in menstrual cycle).

In the proliferative phase, the endometrium is, at first, thin with sparse glands which have straight, narrow lumens. The cervical mucus is scant and viscous. As oestrogen levels rise, secreted by the developing follicle in the ovary, the endometrium thickens three to five times, the glands proliferate and the spiral arterioles elongate. Cervical mucus becomes copious, watery and contains an elastic substance creating channels for sperm entry.

If no conception occurs the secretory phase commences. The progesterone levels rise, under the influence of the growing corpus luteum in the ovary, and endometrial growth stops. Glycogen in the glands moves to their lumen and is secreted in large quantities. The uterus lining becomes oedematous and the arteries elongate and coil. The cervical mucus becomes sticky and reduces in quantity. The arteries go into spasm and release prostaglandins, which ultimately leads to tissue necrosis and cell death in the endometrium. This layer is then shed and menstrual flow occurs. Approximately 50 ml of blood, glandular secretions and tissue fragments flow from the uterine cavity – about two tablespoons. Interestingly, the menstrual blood does not clot until it reaches the vagina because some of the clotting factors normally found in blood are destroyed by the enzymes of the uterus.

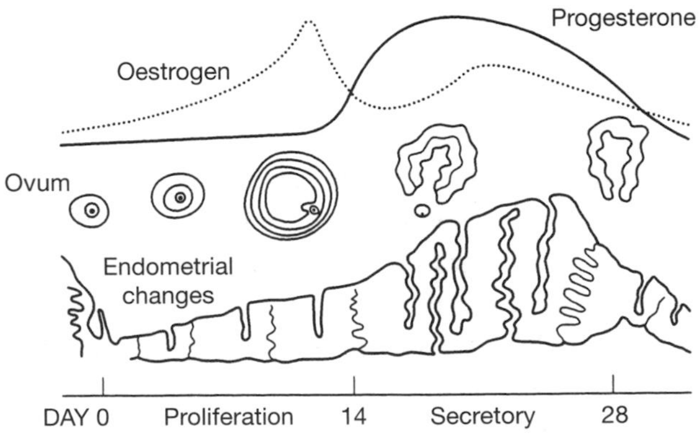

Figure 8.9 Uterine lining, ova changes and circulating hormones during the menstrual cycle

The clots that appear with a heavy flow are a combination of red blood cell clumps, mucus, glycogen and glycoproteins.

Sexually transmitted diseases

Adolescent health (defined as for those between the ages of ten to twelve years by the WHO) has shown no change in the UK for the last twenty years in the area of obesity, smoking, sexually transmitted disease and teenage pregnancy. These problems have been closely linked to risk taking activities such as drinking alcohol, violence, illicit drug taking and sexual intimacy as they 'explore' adult behaviours (Viner and Barker 2005). Tripp and Viner (2005) showed that having unsafe sex for the first time at an early age is often associated with lack of knowledge, lack of access to contraceptives, lack of skill to negotiate use of contraception, and having sex while drunk. This has led to a rise in sexually transmitted diseases such as Chlamydia, which affects 30–40 per cent of sexually active teenage girls. Gonorrhea and genital herpes infections have also increased. However, cultural and socio-economic effects may be influencing the high levels of infection especially among black Caribbean and black African young people. McCance and Heuther (2006) explain how long-term pelvic inflammatory disease, infertility, chronic pelvic pain, neonatal morbidity and genital cancers are the consequences of untreated sexually transmitted conditions and that teenage females are at most risk because of their immature cervix and immunity.

Some simple explanation of the more common conditions is useful for this age group: what the infection is, what the symptoms are and what treatments will work. This information can help them ensure a healthy attitude to sexual behaviour.

- Three bacteria are commonly identified:
  - Chlamydia, *Chlamidia trachomatis*, is the leading cause of infertility;
  - Gonorrhea, *Neisseria gonorrhoeae*;
  - non-specific urethritis (NSU) which is caused by a variety of bacteria.

  All these bacteria infect mucus membranes and cause inflammation of the tissues, pain and exudate – a discharge. Sometimes the discharge is ignored and scarring takes place of the inflamed tissue, which then leads to loss of function of that tissue. All can be successfully treated with antibiotics which eradicate the organism.

- Three viruses are commonly identified:
  - Genital *herpes* which moves to the dorsal sacral nerve root when in the 'resting' phase. It causes painful blisters on the mucus membrane surface. This can be treated with drugs such as aciclovir which disrupts the virus replication but symptoms may return when the child's immune system is compromised such as when stressed or ill (Simonsen *et al.* 2006).
  - *Human papillomavirus* – genital warts. These are very contagious but can disappear spontaneously over time. The problem is that they can be painful but can be treated with topical medications.
  - *Molluscum contagiosum* – a virus of the pox group. It is a benign viral infection often contracted through sharing swimming pool towels. The pearl like warts can spread over the buttocks and perineum and are itchy. They are spread when the child scratches the lesions. They will remain for weeks and sometimes years but are not life threatening, just unsightly and annoying for the child.

- Two parasites are noteworthy:
  - *Trichomoniasis vaginalis* is a protozoa, a one celled organism with a flagellum that swims in the mucus fluid. It causes itching and discharge.
  - *Sarcoptes scabiei – scabes* – is a mite which causes irritation as it burrows into the skin tissues. It is transmitted skin to skin, often when beds are shared.

- One fungus is commonly found by half of all women in their life time – *candida albicans*. This is called vaginal thrush and is NOT a sexually transmitted disease. It is caused by a fungus that normally lives harmlessly round the perineum but invades the vagina when the pH (acidity) changes. This may occur after a course of antibiotics or during pregnancy. The discharge is thick and creamy and the fungus also causes a very uncomfortable irritation because it adheres to the mucus membrane of the vagina and inflames the lining. There are topical treatments that work well but if symptoms continue the cause of the discharge may not be so simple and a visit to a health professional should be encouraged (www.patient.co.uk).

Physiology knowledge in practice

Scenario 1

Sally, aged fifteen years, is having trouble with her 'periods' – they are painful and sometimes make her faint. What is the explanation for these symptoms and how can Sally be helped?

Some pointers:

- This is called dysmenorrhoea: it is the painful menstrual flow caused by chemicals produced during the first forty-eight hours of menstruation. It is often familial so Sally's female relatives may suffer the same symptoms.
- There is the excessive production of endometrial prostaglandin which is a myometrial (uterine muscle) stimulant and vasoconstrictor (closes arterioles in the muscle tissue). This restricts oxygen flow to the muscle cells and causes ischaemia – pain caused due to the death of the cells and the release of potassium from the cell cytoplasm that irritates the pain endings in the intercellular spaces.
- There is also an increase of leukotrines which increase the sensitivity of the pain fibres in the mymetrium.
- There is also an increase in vasopressin which increases ischaemia in the myometrium and makes it hypersensitive.
- There is also pelvic pain, groin pain, backache, loss of appetite that often accompanies the experience of pain, vomiting, diarrhoea, fainting and headaches if the prostaglandins reach the systemic blood stream from the uterus and circulate round the body (www.kidshealth.org).

What can be done?

- Hormonal contraceptives stop this because they stop ovulation and create an atrophic (not engorged with blood vessels ready for conception) endometrium: prostaglandins are not produced and thus do not irritate the myometrium to cause the cramps.
- Prostaglandin inhibitors would work if taken at the start of the bleed/cramping.
- Exercise reduces the symptoms; walking and running are recommended activities.
- Local heat, massage and relaxation techniques help the pain (http://womenshealth.about.com, www.fda.gov).

Scenario 2

Mike and May are thirteen years old and have developed acne. What explanation can you give them on this condition?

The theory

- Spots are common in 85 per cent of the population at this age.
- There may be a genetic family history of acne.
- It is related to a rise in androgens produced in the adrenal cortex in both sexes (also stimulates pubic and axilla hair growth) during early puberty where the sebaceous (oil) glands grow in size and secrete more sebum.
- The bacterium *p. acnes* invades the glands and causes inflammation – the follicle wall (shaft for the hair) breaks down and white cells are attracted from the blood stream through the intercellular spaces to engulf the invasion of bacteria. Pus is formed (dead bacteria and white blood cells).

What can be done?

- Diet is not the cause – chocolate and fatty foods will only produce more adipose tissue when consumed in excess.
- Topical antibiotics are best used and good cleaning regimes of the skin adhered to – do not squeeze and pick them as this will cause scarring later!
- Severe cases can be treated with systemic antibiotics, sex hormones, cortisones and some skin surgery.

Extend your knowledge

Tripp and Viner (2005) suggest that sexual health education is vital to adolescent health in their article 'Sexual health, contraception and teenage pregnancy'. Read this paper and investigate their suggestions as to reasons for unsafe sexual activities in this group and their thoughts on safe sex advice. Extend your own knowledge on drugs that are used by teenagers and how pregnancy may be the outcome for both thoughtless male and female behaviour.

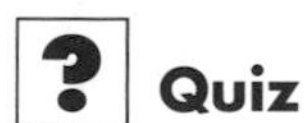

A – hormone that starts the axilla and pubic hair growth
B – the larche is the development of what
C – we have forty-six of these in every cell other than the gonads
D – the vas ***** allows sperm to move from the testes to the penis in ejaculation
E – lining of the uterus
F – name of the tube through which the egg moves to the uterus from the ovary
G – section of the chromosome responsible for an individual trait
H – chemical that is released from an endocrine gland – GnRH is one
I – canal in the abdominal wall that the testes move through to reach the scrotum
J – the pre-pubescent immature state
K – a route of disease transmission much loved by teenagers to show affection
L – produce testosterone
M – the start of menstruation
N – the homeostatic balance that stops the hypothalamus producing GnRH
O – where eggs are stored and matured
P – a time of reproductive maturation

Now you can complete the alphabet for yourself.

Chapter 9

The immune system

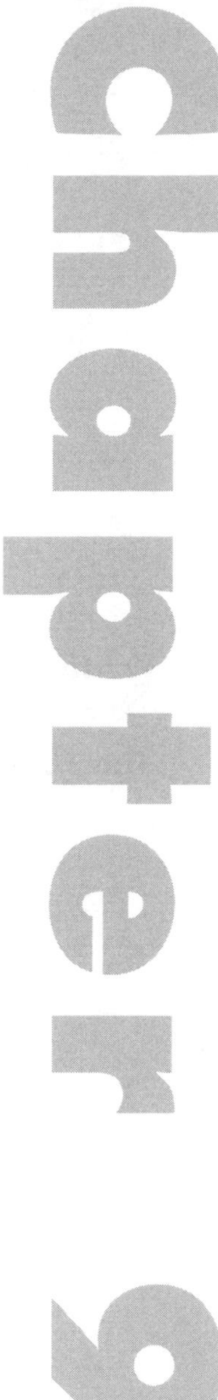

- Protection from micro-organisms – the three lines of defence
- Lymphocyte development in the embryo
- Immunoglobulin (Ig) production in the foetus and newborn
- The rhesus factor
- Embryology of the thymus gland and T lymphocyte development
- Lymph vessel development
- Stress
- The damaging chronic stress hormones
- Resilience
- The physiology of immunisation
- Points of interest when vaccinating children

INFANTS AND CHILDREN are susceptible to attack from the micro-environment, as their immune systems require many years to develop. Before birth the foetus is protected, to a large extent, by its mother's defences and the placenta. Resistance to infection thereafter depends on general body defence mechanisms, innate genetic inheritance and an acquired passive or active resistance from their ongoing exposure to the world around them. Internal and external stressors can reduce their resistance to disease; immunisation programmes (see Chapter 1) aim to boost their ability to remain healthy and thus allow them to develop to their optimum physical condition. Protection from micro-organisms is provided by a series of 'barriers'.

Protection from micro-organisms – the three lines of defence

The first line of defence – the skin

Intact skin and mucosa surfaces act as the primary non-immunological host defence, the first line defence (see Figure 9.1). The antimicrobial enzyme, lysozyme, which helps to breakdown the polysaccharide cell wall of gram positive bacteria, is present in secretions such as sweat, tears and saliva. The acidity of gastric juices will usually kill ingested bacteria but is less efficient in the very young. Other 'protective' activities such as cilia movement in the upper respiratory

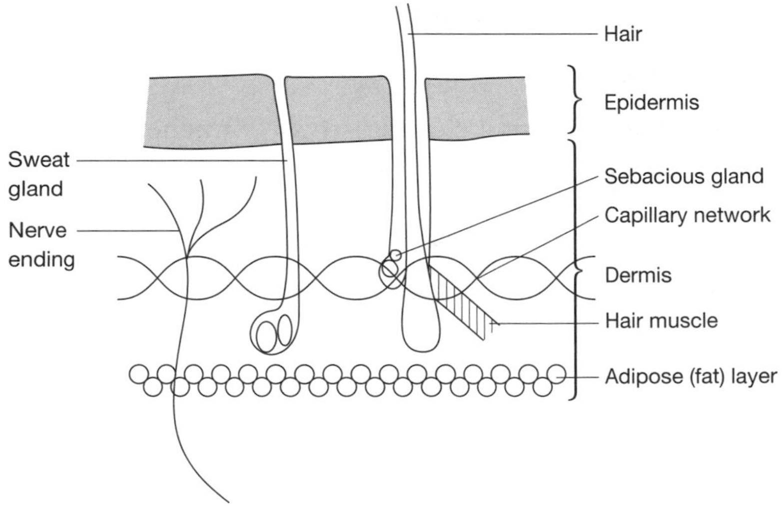

Figure 9.1 Skin

tract that sweeps particles to the pharynx and 'friendly' bacteria in the gut, such as *e.coli* and *lactobacillus* in the vagina and urinary tract of females, also provide barriers to invasion (see previous chapters for revision).

The second line of defence – inflammation, white blood cells and the immune response

Inflammation is a normal protective reaction to harmful organisms entering the body or other cell insults (see Figure 9.2 for protective inflammatory reaction). It is a complex reaction that involves white blood cells, platelets and mast cells which contain the chemical histamine that resides near blood capillaries. It results in the vascular and cell changes that respond to protect the cell further injury due to infection, mechanical damage, ischemia (lack of oxygen supply), lack of nutrients, immune defects such as those of children who are given cancer therapy, chemical agents, temperature extremes such as high fever or frost bite, and radiation such as sunburn. The chemicals which trigger these events are derived from both specific tissue cells and circulating plasma proteins. It can be observed both locally and systemically. An inflamed area will look red, hot, sore, swollen and with a watery or pus filled exudate (see Figure 9.3 for inflammatory vascular response). The child may also have a fever as the chemicals

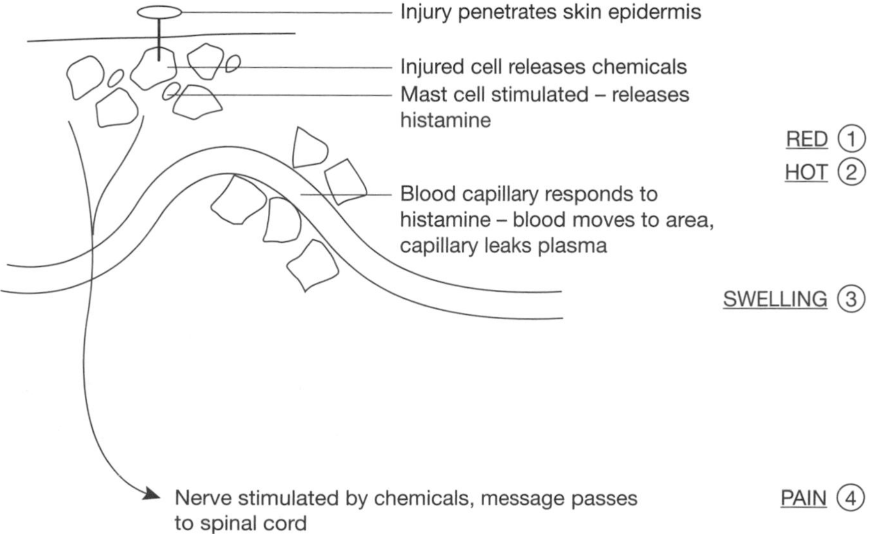
Injury penetrates skin epidermis
Injured cell releases chemicals
Mast cell stimulated – releases histamine
RED ①
HOT ②
Blood capillary responds to histamine – blood moves to area, capillary leaks plasma
SWELLING ③
Nerve stimulated by chemicals, message passes to spinal cord
PAIN ④

Figure 9.2 Inflammation reaction in skin

stimulate the hypothalamus to raise the body temperature and disrupt the antigen multiplying. Contemporary practice is to allow the child's temperature to reach 38 °C before antipyretics are offered in order to support this natural defence mechanism. However, neonates will need a more speedy intervention as they have an immature chemical production ability; they are more vulnerable to invasions and have a weaker inflammation response.

The white cells of the blood that are active in the inflammation response are derived from bone marrow precursor cells (stem cells). They can multiply if stimulated by repeated exposure to antigens (invading organisms) in the blood or tissues. Blood cells differentiate from two types of bone marrow stem cells, the myeloid and the lymphoid. The myeloid cells differentiate to six types of cell. The first type are platelets, which are important for blood clotting. The second type are red blood cells, important for oxygen transport. The third type are monocytes which grow to phagocytes, important for 'eating' dead tissue and invading organisms. The fourth type, the neutrophils, form an integral part of the immune system and are the most common white blood cells, destroying bacteria. The fifth type are eosinophils, being active in parasitic infection and the final type, basophils, are important in the inflammatory response.The lymphoid type cells differentiate between T cells via the thymus gland responsible for virus attack and B cells via the liver and bone marrow itself responsible for bacterial attack (Playfair and Chain 2001). These

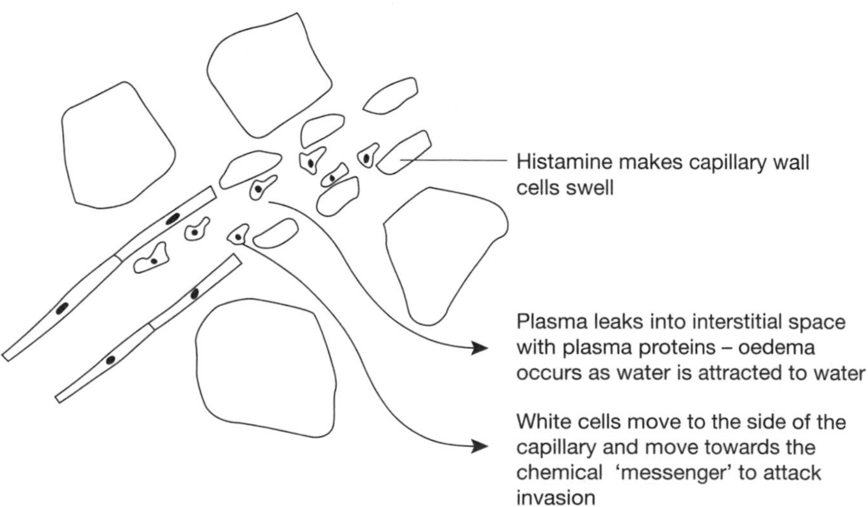
Histamine makes capillary wall cells swell
Plasma leaks into interstitial space with plasma proteins – oedema occurs as water is attracted to water
White cells move to the side of the capillary and move towards the chemical 'messenger' to attack invasion

Figure 9.3 Vascular response in inflammation

B lymphocyte cells make antibodies – chemicals that destroy invaders. Another name for an antibody is an immunoglobulin (Ig). Immunoglobulins are proteins; they are classified as M, G, A, E and D. IgG is the most abundant, making up 75 per cent of the total antibody population. It crosses the placenta and gives the foetus its natural passive immunity. IgA is present in our mucus membranes and tears; it protects out respiratory tract and conjunctiva which are constantly exposed to external attack from airborne particles. IgE is produced in allergic reactions and can cause us harm by excessive stimulation of inflammation of local tissue such as a response to eating peanuts. The exact function of IgD is not well understood.

There are also three chemical cascades that are stimulated via the blood proteins when cell damage occurs: complement which is stimulated by the antigen being attacked by the antibody (chemical produced by the B lymphocytes), clotting which is stimulated by damage to the blood capillary lining, and kinin which unlocks bradekinin, a chemical which supports the action of prostaglandins released by damaged cell membranes to start the inflammatory process.

The immune response (see Figure 9.4) relies on communication with all other cellular defence systems through a network of chemical messengers called cytokines. However, the principal cells are the lymphocytes which are mobile cells found in the blood, lymph nodes, spleen and tissue spaces. Lymphocytes can usually discriminate between self and non-self cells; however, sometimes this can go wrong and 'autoimmune' conditions occur where they attack body cells such as in arthritis. They require interaction with the macrophages – the big eaters – which alert the lymphocytes by secreting cytokines and 'eat' the destroyed invader.

The third line of defence – acquisition of immunity

Immunity is acquired in two ways. Active immunity follows exposure and stimulation of the immune response to any infection, such as the common cold and chickenpox, or by immunisation against hepatitis, measles, mumps and rubella (MMR). In this situation, the lymphocytes 'remember' the 'shape' of the invading antigen by altering their cell walls so that when the antigen is contacted again it can multiply quickly to produce the antibodies to eradicate the foreign protein. Sometimes this process of experiencing an invasion is considered dangerous, so immunisation can speed the process up by

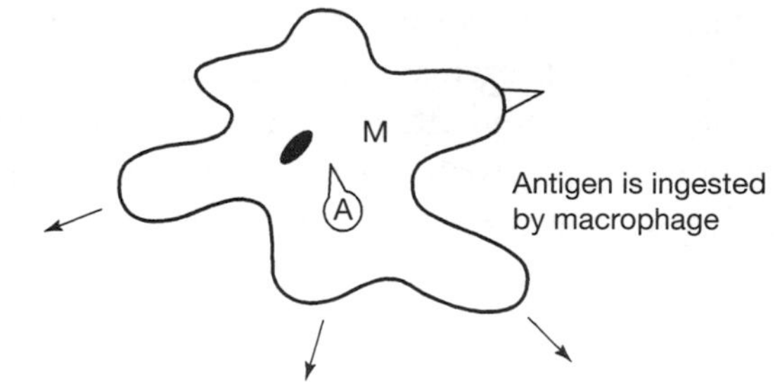
M
A
Antigen is ingested by macrophage
Secretes monokine chemical

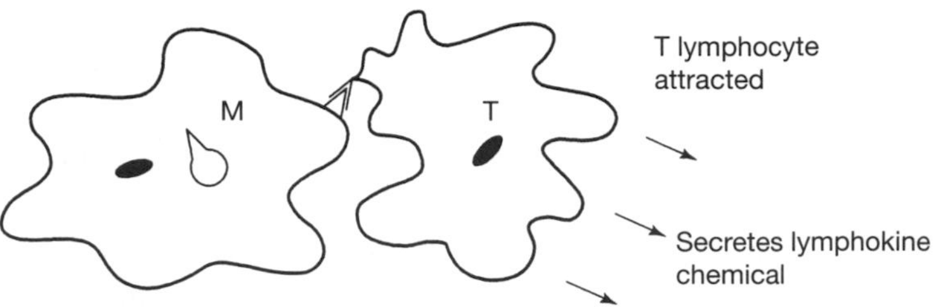
M
T
T lymphocyte attracted
Secretes lymphokine chemical

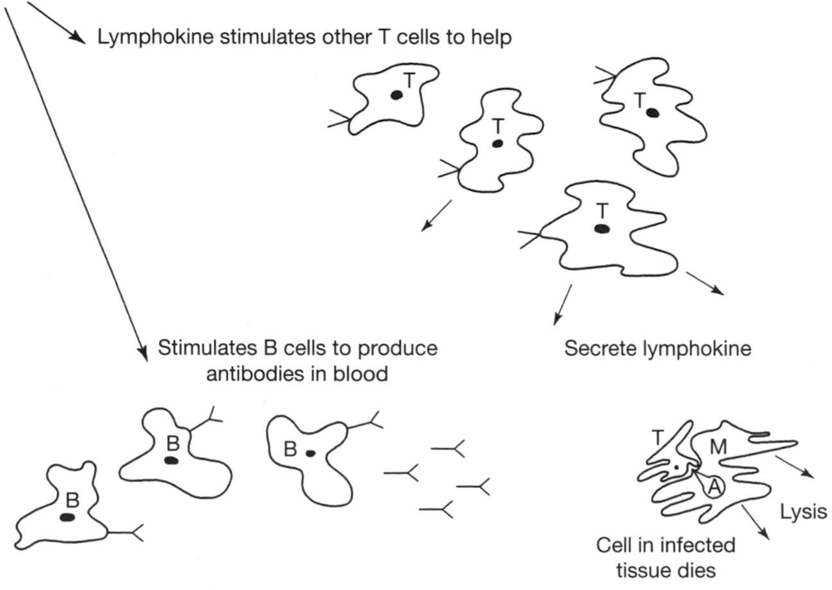
Lymphokine stimulates other T cells to help
T
T
T
T
Secrete lymphokine
Stimulates B cells to produce antibodies in blood
B
B
B
T
M
A
Lysis
Cell in infected tissue dies

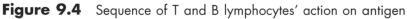

Figure 9.4 Sequence of T and B lymphocytes' action on antigen

injections of 'weakened' antigen to stimulate a response before the infection is experienced – an example is the measles vaccine. Passive immunity is short-lived immunity, occurring when Igs are passed to the individual, such as when the mother passes her protection to the foetus across the placenta, to her baby in breast milk, or when they are injected into immuno-compromised children who have not been immunised or lost their immunity and are exposed to viruses such as chickenpox when they are very ill (Playfair and Chain 2001).

Lymphocyte development in the embryo

The development of the lymphocytes in the foetus show that the premature baby will be at risk from any environment, as will the newborn, who is not immediately immunised. There are two types of lymphocytes: B and T.

B cells

B cells appear in the liver a week later than T cells are identifiable. They then migrate to the bone marrow. B cells in the foetal liver differ from those found later in the bone marrow. Earlier cells make Igs (antibodies) that can bind to a wide variety of antigens but with relatively low affinity. The later cells make antibodies that react more strongly with their specific antigen nearer the time of birth. In the bone marrow interleukin binds to receptors on the pro B and pre B cells, signalling them to divide and differentiate. First, they encode their genetic fragments to form Igs, they then grow antigen receptors on their cell surfaces which will respond to foreign invasion. However, immature B cells cannot differentiate spontaneously; they need nearby mature B cells to donate their molecular message (genetic fragments) before they can themselves mature and be released into the bloodstream. Complete B cells are needed to make subsequent generations. This development appears to be genetically programmed, as they need no antigen stimulus for this activity. Over the period of a lifetime, potentially ninety years of constant interaction with millions of invading antigens in the bloodstream, B cells will be capable of much change in order to protect the individual by identifying the ever increasing variety of invaders. B cells secrete a number of Igs (antibodies):

- Between 5 and 10 per cent are IgA, which has a half life of seven days. IgA is concentrated in the respiratory and gastrointestinal (GI) tract, for example, in saliva, tears and GI secretions. It attaches to exposed tissue surfaces by combining with a component from their epithelial cells. Breastfed babies appear to be protected from intestinal infection early in life by this antibody.
- IgG is the major Ig found in the lymphoid tissues; it represents 75 per cent of all Igs and has the smallest structure. It recognises micro-organisms and activates complement. It passes from blood to interstitial spaces, and moves easily through the placenta to provide the foetus and newborn with maternally acquired immunity for the first three months of life. It is present in high concentrations in colostrum and breast milk. Interestingly, some cultural groups advocate the disposal of colostrum before the mother's milk 'comes in' for their newborn babies – the reason for this may not be physiological.
- IgE is the Ig involved in allergic, anaphylactic and atopic reactions. The allergic individual responds to antigen invasion by combining the allergen with IgE rather than IgG, thus it is not phagocytosed. The IgE/antigen complex, instead, then stimulates mast cells in the tissues to produce histamine. Allergens such as pollen, certain foods, drugs, dust, insect venom, moulds and animal dander can produce this effect. IgE levels are raised in sensitised children.
- IgM comprises 10 per cent of the Igs and stays in the bloodstream. It is a large molecule which reacts with foreign antigens in the blood. It also activates complement and is the major Ig produced in infancy.

Immunoglobulin (Ig) production in the foetus and newborn

B cells that synthesise IgM appear first, followed by those destined to make IgG. B lymphocytes, able to make IgA, appear to a limited extent near the time of birth. The numbers of these three Igs, M, G and A, in the foetus are low unless the unborn baby is exposed to antigens; then the presence of IgM may be seen to rise in the blood as early as twenty-eight weeks' gestation. However, it is IgG that is transported across the placenta to the greatest extent; therefore, this is the normal Ig profile of the newborn, even though the foetus only contributes about 5 per cent to this number. After birth, these levels give protection to the baby for the first few months of life while the baby's own production rises. Premature infants may be deficient in IgG because most is transferred in the last trimester. However, the transfer of these Igs depends on the structural and functional aspects of the placenta as well as the receptor-mediated mechanism. The rate and selectivity of their transfer is also influenced by the ability of the foetal capillary endothelial cells and trophoblasts covering the chorionic villi to transport these protein structures without changing their shape. These IgG reach adult levels, eventually, by four years old. This may explain the young child's vulnerability to infections.

The rhesus factor

Rhesus isoimmunisation occurs when the foetus red cells carry rhesus positive antigen and the mother is rhesus negative. As foetal red cells can always enter the blood of the mother, the mother develops Igs against them of the IgM then IgG class. These IgG antibodies are then transported to the foetus and clump foetal red cells to destroy them. This reaction is 'sensitised' by the first pregnancy, but more destructive in subsequent pregnancies as the mother responds more quickly after her body has 'learnt' to recognise this foreign structure.

Embryology of the thymus gland and T lymphocyte development

The thymus is vital for the maturation of the T lymphocyte and is only evident in childhood. By the end of adolescence it has shrivelled and is non-functioning. Thereafter, T cells clone themselves (reproduce by mitosis – see Chapter 8 for explanation) in the lymph glands when required to fight viral infections. Children often have swollen glands in the neck when they have 'colds'; HIV (human immunodeficiency virus) is a devastating infection that destroys these vital white blood cells and renders the individual lethally exposed to the micro-environment because they have no mechanisms for replacing them if they are totally destroyed.

In embryonic development of the throat, four pharyngeal pouches separate the branchial arches in the pharyngeal part of the foregut.

The endoderm lining of the pouch's dorsal end then gives rise to the inferior parathyroid glands, whereas the ventral part gives rise to the thymus gland. In the sixth gestational week, the third pharyngeal pouch pinches off from the pharynx. In weeks seven and eight, the thymic primordia, one each side, elongate and migrate caudally. As the thymus epithelium proliferates, the two thymic primordia develop from hollow tubes to solid glands. By week eight, these fuse medially (Figure 9.5). The thymus in the neonate is of a variable shape with either no lobulations, or appears bilobar or trilobar, and is located finally in the mediastinum.

The thymus has two functions. The first is differentiation of primitive lymphocytes, which have migrated from the bone marrow into immuno-competent T cells. They pass to the thymus before seeding (moving) to the lymph tissues of the body over several days. T cells differentiate into many different T cells in the thymus. Here they are presented with antigens by mature cells, to which they must react in order to survive. As they mature, they may reorganise their genes to produce T cell receptors on their membrane surfaces and thus become killer cells or helper/suppressor cells for B lymphocytes. By gestational week nine, lymphocytes appear in the lymph and blood systems, thus the immune system is developed early in intra-uterine life. By the fifteenth week about 65 per cent of the lymphocytes in the foetal thymus are T cells.

The second role of the thymus is the further expansion of antigen-stimulating T cells by the production of extracts or hormonal substances such as thymosin. T cells help in the attack on bacterial,

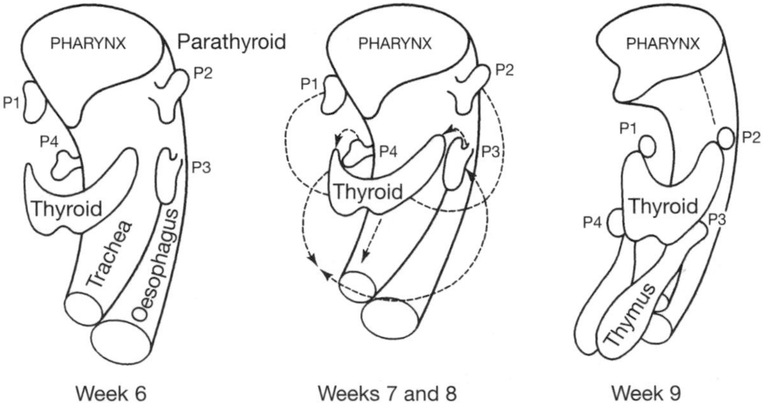

Figure 9.5 Thymus development

viral, parasitic and mycotic micro-organisms, they are responsible for the auto-immune phenomena, and they also participate in the rejection of malignant and transplanted cells (McCance and Heuther 2006).

Lymph vessel development

The lymph system includes a wide network of collecting vessels and ducts that permeate most organs. It is the main way that white blood cells are circulated in the body to provide protection from invasion from the micro-environment immune response. Unlike the cardiovascular loop system, it is an open ended one way system. It assists in maintaining the blood volume by collecting fluid, wastes and white blood cells that are in excess in the interstitial spaces. Its glands hold white blood cells ready for action when an invasion of antigens occurs. Its vessels have 'blind' endings that open as tissue pressure builds up, a tissue pump. This excess fluid is then moved up through the body to empty into the returning large veins at the base of the neck, to the heart (see Figure 9.6, blind ending of lymph vessel in interstitial space). They are, like blood capillaries, made of a single endothelial

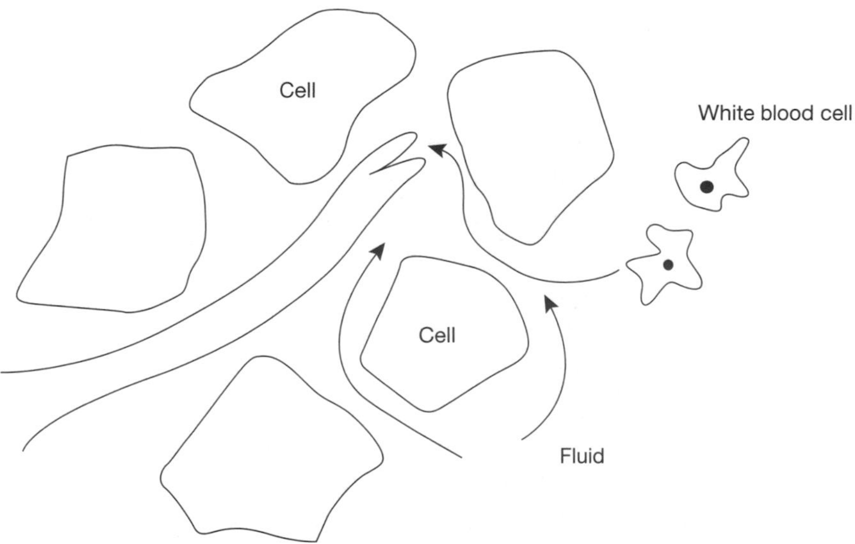

As pressure builds in spaces between cells the vessel ending opens to allow excess fluid and white blood cells to enter

Figure 9.6 Lymph vessel blind ending

layer of cells but have a wider lumen, have well formed valves to stop backflow and are firmly adhered to the surrounding connective tissue. Thus, they are very sensitive to tissue stress such as increased fluid retention (Scavelli *et al.* 2004).

The lymph vessels develop in the fifth and sixth week after conception, in a similar way to the venous blood capillaries. Early lymph vessels sprout from embryo veins and grow into surrounding tissues and organs where the lymphatic vessels grow. These small tubes join together to form a closed network of vessels and lymph sacs. The six major lymph sacs are two jugular in the neck, two iliac in the groin, a retroperitoneal in the abdomen, and one cisterna chyli in the chest which drains into the venous circulation at the junction of the internal jugular and subclavian veins. There are many smaller lymph nodes in the body; children with sore throats often experience their swelling in the neck, or behind the knee if they damage their foot. This lymphatic system is present at birth.

Stress

Stress can mean different things to different individuals and children are no different. However, the physiological changes are common to all stress reactions. Stress is important for motivation – a state of eustress where the body is prepared for action; however, too much stimulus is distressing and it is this distress that can be physiologically measured and is the cause of much eventual illness. The immune system is the most profoundly affected system of the body by the hormones released by the adrenal cortex during chronic stress. Stress is possibly a natural consequence of all children's lifestyles today, and to some extent immune deficiency will result from their exposure to chronic stressors that they perceive to be threatening. One must remember that children may see things as stressful which are not obviously so to adults; it is then the way that individual children deal with particular situations that may cause their immune system to become compromised. Stressors can be many things for them, such as recurrent infections from repeated tonsillitis, chaotic home life or school worries.

The adrenal medulla and adrenal cortex have complementary roles in promoting a widespread adaptation to stress; a coordinated adaptive response where the adrenal medulla initially secretes adrenaline in response to an initial fear, stimulated by the brain's perception of danger which is then mediated by the adrenal cortex's increased secretion of cortisol as the frightening situation extends (Marieb and Hoehn 2007).

In 'acute' stress, the cortex of the brain perceives a threatening situation and activates the autonomic nervous system sympathetic branch via the hypothalamus to release adrenaline and noradrenaline from the chromaffin cells in the adrenal medulla. These hormones circulate in the blood to prepare the body for flight. The child will look pale, sweaty and have raised alertness; metabolic rate will rise and heart rate and breathing will increase (Figure 9.7).

If the stressful situation continues, the hypothalamus activates a second system which affects the pituitary gland and its release of prolactin, growth hormone, endorphins and adrenocorticotropic hormone (ACTH), which stimulate the adrenal cortex to secrete cortisol (Figure 9.8).

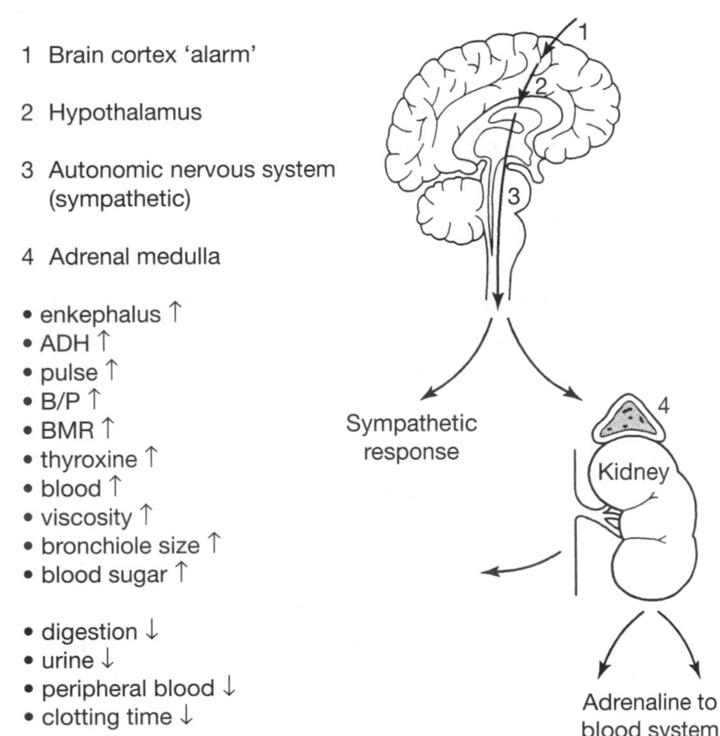

Figure 9.7 The 'acute' stress response

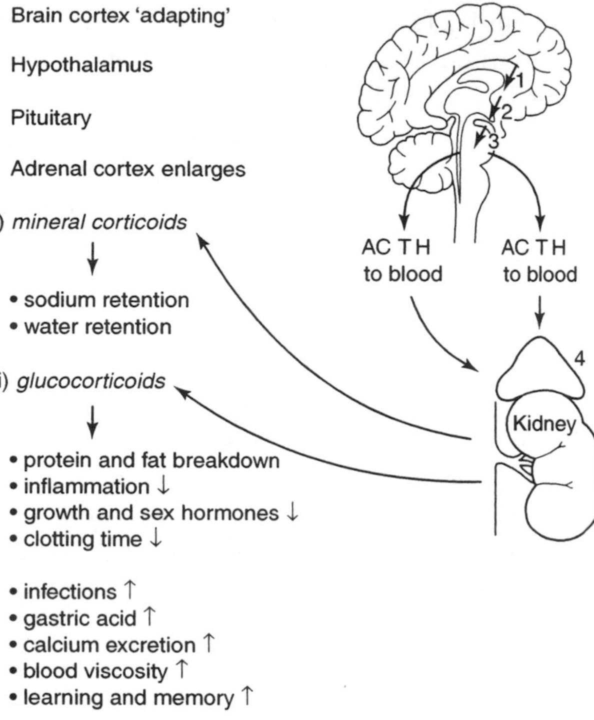

Figure 9.8 The 'chronic' stress response

The damaging chronic stress hormones

Chronic stress is damaging to the physical growth and development of children; the chemical of stress will leave them exposed to a reduced response to the micro-environment and may be the cause of disabling symptoms – constant tummy ache, headaches, weight gain/loss and mood changes. The hypothalamus/pituitary and adrenal endocrine hormones have a variety of known effects:

- Cortisol from the adrenal cortex acts as an immunosuppressant by reducing protein synthesis, including the blood immunoglobins. It reduces peripheral blood eosinophils, lymphocytes and macrophages. Large amounts of cortisol promote atrophy of the lymphoid tissue in the thymus, spleen and lymph nodes, thus reducing T cell production. It directly reduces the immune response to antigens; infections will be more easily able to gain entry to the body. It also inhibits the production of interleukin, one from the macrophages and interleukin and two from the helper T cells.

It reduces the T and B cell response to antigen challenges and the generation of fever by the complement cascade. However, it can promote increased energy levels as the breakdown of protein releases sugar into the blood for muscle activity and amino-acids for creation of new tissue. Cortisol increases gastric acid secretion and may disrupt the female menstrual cycle.

- Endorphins, secreted with ACTH in chronic stress situations, come from the pituitary and central nervous system. They regulate the production of ACTH, produce a reduced sensitivity to pain and a raised feeling of excitement. One could ask whether it is this chemical that allows children to become 'numb' and distance themselves from frightening circumstances, or those children who appear shy or are easily excitable. This may be how they 'cope' when they have no way of escape from their situation.
- Growth hormone, produced by the pituitary gland, rises after the stress of physical exercise, and also with psychological stimulus. Children who are active, interested and sleep well will grow. However, growth hormone is also stimulated by watching violent films and playing violent games. For each individual child there will be a point when excitement turns into distress and reduces the production of this hormone. When this happens, lymphocyte function is disrupted and the immune response becomes less effective.
- Prolactin, also secreted from the pituitary, acts as a second messenger for interleukin 2, and normally increases B cell activation and differentiation. It is reduced in prolonged stress, especially from physical injury. Children are therefore vulnerable to this stressor as they are more prone to accidents at all ages.

Resilience

Children's responses to stress begin pre-natally and develop more fully as the child interacts with the environment. Their response to any stressor is individual; some children are more adaptive than others. Many experts now recognise the different levels of resilience that can be found in all children regardless of their social/emotional situation (Bee and Boyd 2007, www.scotland.gov.uk, Stevenson 2007) and suggest that the child's individual disposition, family warmth and having positive models to identify with are important in learning coping strategies. They describe resilience as 'the ability to bounce back' in the face of adversity; to know how and where and from whom to get support when problems arise. They suggest that children with above average IQ, an easy going temperament, who are attractive and in good health, have all the attributes to cope with life. Carers of children can support and develop this capability to a smaller or larger degree in all children by being a good role model, having a trusting and caring relationship with the young people, giving them a sense of mastery over the tasks they asked to perform, instilling self confidence, helping them to manage their feelings, respond to feelings of others and develop a sense of humour (www.healthpromoting schools.co.uk).

Each child requires the carer to respond to unique cues: demanding behaviour, failure to attain 'milestones' and failure to thrive are signs of stress in the very young. The pre-school child may become incontinent, have night terrors and become aggressive. The school-aged child may refuse to go to school and fall behind in studies. The adolescent may worry about his or her changing body, heightened sexuality, peer pressure and parental discord. Challenges that are appropriate, such as encouraging particular interests and success in sport for the adolescent, will stimulate the child to move on to the next stage of their physical competence. Inappropriate stressors, such as the need to achieve in school examinations beyond their competence or towards others' goals, will result in a slower and more dysfunctional development.

The physiology of immunisation

By 2007 many communicable diseases have become rare, and the resulting morbidity and mortality reduced. Vaccination programmes have traditionally been a national responsibility; however, with the advent of new vaccines for many of the less devastating infections, such as mumps, parents need to be properly informed rather than morally cajoled before they present their offspring for more and more recommended injections. In the USA, children cannot access education without their vaccinations being up to date, yet in the UK where vaccination is free, not all children are protected. There is information freely available and there is no charge for the service in the UK (www. immunization.nhs.uk, www.patient.co.uk, www.direct.gov.uk).

Vaccination stimulates the immune system in a variety of ways without the need for the individual to suffer the condition:

- Live but weakened (attenuated) pathogenic micro-organisms stimulate the body to recognise a foreign (antigen) protein and produce antibodies to destroy it. The memory created protects the child from future invasion of the particular pathogen. MMR vaccine can induce a mild form of measles within ten days of vaccination and/or a general inflammatory response.
- Dead organisms can be injected which have the 'shape' of the antigen but cannot divide and multiply in the body. The lymphocytes recognise them as foreign and respond, again producing a memory cell of the 'shape' for future attacks. Typhoid and pertussis (whooping cough) are commonly used in vaccination programmes. A new acellular vaccine for pertussis is available which, it is hoped, will produce a less severe reaction yet give protection from future infection.
- Toxoids, such as those from tetanus and diphtheria, are the modified bacterial toxin that has been made non-toxic, but which retains the ability to stimulate the formation of antibodies.

For details on the recommended UK immunisation schedule, see Chapter 1 and www.immunization.nhs.uk.

Points of interest when vaccinating children

- If a viral vaccine is to be used, it will not be effective if the child has a viral infection such as the common cold. Inferon will be present in the bloodstream, which will inhibit the body's response to the vaccine.
- If oral polio vaccine is given to a child with a gastrointestinal infection such as diarrhoea and vomiting, the vaccine will be passed out of the gut and not completely absorbed. Even after successful polio vaccination, children will 'shed' the virus in their faeces for six weeks.
- Some viruses are cultured for vaccines in egg tissue with antibiotics that suppress bacterial contamination. Some children may be hypersensitive and produce an allergic response to these foreign proteins, and release histamine into the tissues.

- The measles vaccine is given after one year, as the residual maternal IgG will destroy the organism before it has elicited a response. The measles vaccine activates the immune system in a non-specific way which provides protection against other diseases. However, there continues to be publicity speculating that this particular vaccine is responsible for children developing Crohn's disease and autism, which is not currently supported by research.

Physiology knowledge in practice

Scenario 1

Stuart, aged sixteen years, has a persistent cough and cold. He has recently completed his examinations and has been on an adventure holiday with his school friends for two weeks. What could explain this situation and what could be done?

Some pointers:

- Stuart may have chronic stress; cortisol levels are raised due to hard work for some months in preparation for the exams and then the strenuous exercise and little sleep on his holiday. This hormone has released energy from protein stores to allow continuous physical activity.
- His white cell count is low and cannot rid him of the low grade infection.

What can be done?

- Rest and sleep – how could this help him recover his immune response?
- Good nutrition will replenish his nutrient stores – which ones would you suggest are important for the immune system and for an adolescent boy?
- Interesting outdoor activities will keep his brain active – how else could this help?
- A nurturing environment – what could be meant by this?

Scenario 2

Jessie, aged seven years, appears to be allergic to pollen in the spring of each year. What is the physiology for her symptoms of sneezing, blocked nose and weeping eyes and what can be done for her to make things more comfortable at this time of year?

The theory

- Allergy is hypersensitivity to an invading antigen; it is an altered immune response to an allergen.
- Jessie may come from a family who are atopic; they are predisposed to produce more IgE and may suffer asthma, eczema, hay fever or food allergy. Jessie is sensitive to an inhaled stimulus.
- The most common allergies are IgE mediated where repeated exposure to the allergen encourages the IgE to bind to mast cells and produce an inflammatory response.
- The mast cells below the mucus membrane in her upper respiratory tract have released histamine into the tissue of the tract lining. Histamine increases vascular permeability and fluid moves to the interstitial spaces caused swelling – her nose is blocked and keeps her sneezing and blowing her nose to expel secretions.
- The histamine stimulates the prostaglandins released from the damaged cells to irritate the pain nerve endings – her nose and throat are itchy and sore.
- The complement system may be stimulated to raise the body temperature and increase the histamine effect – she feels hot and miserable.

What can be done?

- Anti-histamines are available 'over the counter' at pharmacies. These will reduce histamine effect.
- She could have sensitivity testing at her local hospital to identify the triggers – it may not be only pollen (www.allergyuk.org, http://hcd2.bupa.co.uk).
- She could have de-sensitising treatment for her particular allergen.

Extend your knowledge

Montgomery *et al.* (2006) investigated the histories of 8,958 ten-year-old children in the UK who had divorced parents. They hypothesised that those who had been breastfed would suffer less chronic anxiety – that their adverse exposure would be modified by this early maternal contact. Read their paper 'Breast feeding and resilience against psychosocial stress', and find out what the experiences were which enabled them as babies to modify their neuro-endocrine systems and develop resilience to chronic stress.

? Quiz

1 How is the body protected from infection?
2 What is the body's first line of defence?
3 What causes inflammation?
4 To what cells does the lymphoid bone marrow differentiate?
5 What is active immunity?
6 What is IgE?
7 Which immunoglobulin is transported across the placenta to the greatest extent?
8 What happens when the foetus is damaged by the rhesus factor?
9 Why is the thymus gland important in childhood?
10 What is the main role of the thymus gland?
11 What does the lymph system do?
12 What do the lymph vessels do?
13 What physiological response occurs in the acute stress response?
14 What happens in the body if a stressful situation continues?
15 What effect does cortisol have on the gastric secretions?
16 Define resilience.
17 What can a carer of children do to promote resilience?

18 Explain how a live vaccine works.

19 What is a toxoid?

20 Why may some children show an allergic reaction to vaccination?

Chapter 10

Body and mind

- The limbic area of the brain
- The hypothalamus
- The developing mind

THE INTERACTION OF BOTH nature and nurture in the development of the healthy child underpins their ability to function in their social group. Genetic inheritance 'sets the scene' and physiological maturation determines the healthy child's ability to use the environmental to hone their inbuilt 'experience processing' skills. We infer this process by observing their behaviour and psychologists have documented this activity to suggest developmental 'norms'. They have shown that the brain is more than the electrical impulses that can be measured; consciousness encompasses perception of senses, voluntary initiation and control of movement, and capabilities associated with higher mental processing such as perception, memory, learning and emotional response. Marieb and Hoehn (2007) describes clinical consciousness on a continuum that grades behaviour in response to stimulus as alert, drowsy, stupor and coma, but a wider definition of consciousness, such as that which allows the child to appreciate beauty and experience love, must involve a more holistic and totally interconnected function of brain parts.

The limbic area of the brain

This chapter starts by focusing on the anatomy and physiology of one of the functional areas of the brain, the limbic system, which is derived from the primitive rhin-encephalon 'smell brain'. This is the 'emotional brain' which has extensive connections with lower and higher brain regions allowing integration and response to environmental stimuli. The important structures are the amygdala and hippocampus. The amygdale is responsible for assessing danger and initiating a fear response, whereas the hippocampus is active in memory storing. Much of the output from the limbic area is directed through the hypothalamus, thus an anatomical connection can be seen between emotion response and physical effect as the hypothalamus coordinates all the autonomic nervous and endocrine responses, such as response to stress (in Chapter 9). Because the limbic area also connects to the brain cortex where conscious understanding occurs (the thinking brain), an emotional reaction to understanding can be explained as can the understanding of an emotional response.

Slee and Shute (2003) use this knowledge to suggest an explanation of the neurodevelopment which might result in children developing violent behaviour. Humans evolved as social animals and their

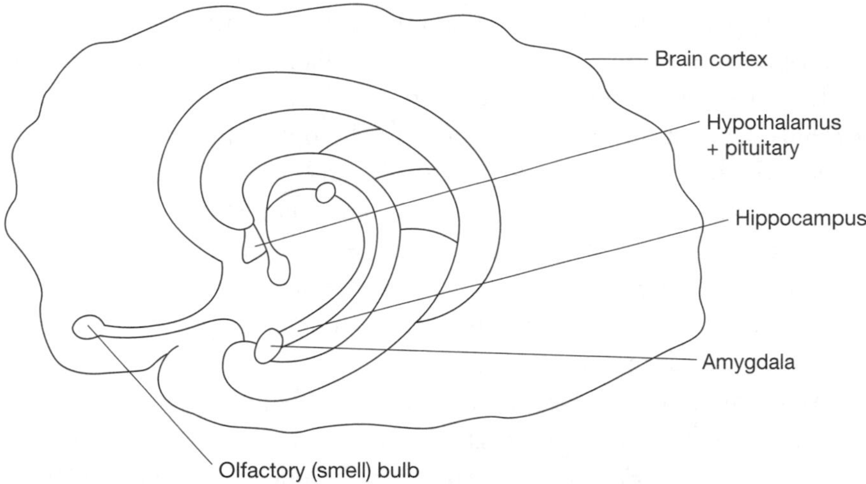

Figure 10.1 The limbic system in the brain

individual survival depended on nurturing the clan. Their cortical development (understanding of situations) modulated the lower parts of the brain such as the mid-brain and limbic area (emotional response). They suggest that if the lower levels of brain development became disrupted the higher levels were less able to control (self control) inappropriate behaviour. They propose that children who are neglected throughout their early years, when the emotional brain is maturing, will result in a child with chronic raised anxiety levels. This can then predispose them to violence because their thinking brain, which matures at a slower rate, will be less able to allow them to maintain self control when situations make them angry or frustrated.

The hypothalamus

The tiny hypothalamus (see Figure 10.1), which is the size of a walnut, is the visceral control centre for the body; there are few functions of the body in which it is not involved. It works through a negative feedback system to maintain homeostasis (physiological balance). It controls the endocrine glands, the autonomic nervous system (sympathetic and parasympathetic branches), body temperature, food intake, water balance and sleep/wake cycles, and is at the centre of the limbic area (Marieb and Hoehn 2007).

The hypothalamus develops from the same structure as the cerebral hemispheres and olfactory tracts. The thalamus and hypothalamus differentiate by the end of the sixth gestational week, the pituitary extends beneath them and lies close to the optic chiasma and pineal gland which are involved in sleep/wake and other biological cycles (Figure 10.2). Many children need 'blackout blinds' in summer when the main external cue for sleep, daylight, extends beyond their normal bed time and internal physiological cues, such as the rise in blood melatonin (the chemical produced by the pineal gland to induce sleepiness) levels, are disrupted.

An example of its coordinating function of emotional and physiological function is in the stress response and the female ovary and menstrual cycles (Figure 10.3). In stressed females, the hypothalamic function of corticotropin-releasing hormone (CRH) activates the adreno-cortico-trophic hormone (ACTH) and inhibits gonadotropin-releasing hormone, growth hormone and sexual activity. The glucocorticoids released in the stress response suppress leutinising hormone and thus ovulation, reduce the production of ovarian oestrogen and progesterone, and render target cells resistant to oestradiol. Teenage girls may then present with amenorrhagia if they are anxious about exams, worried about their social life or unsure of their relationship with parents and family. Absence of periods may also result from the physiological stress of body tissue changes, for example when building

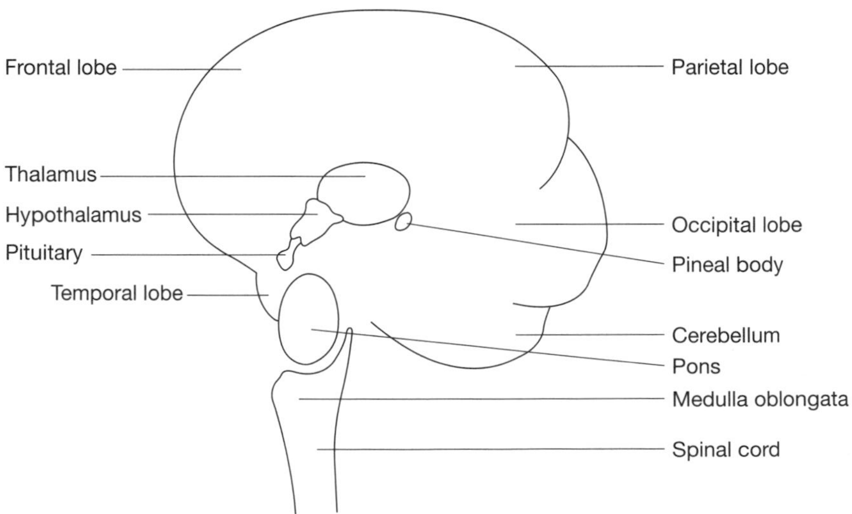

Figure 10.2 Position in brain of thalamus, hypothalamus and pituitary

muscles while training in a particular sport activity such as gymnastics or swimming, or reduction in total body weight when a young person develops anorexia. Pregnancy, however, may need to be discounted first!

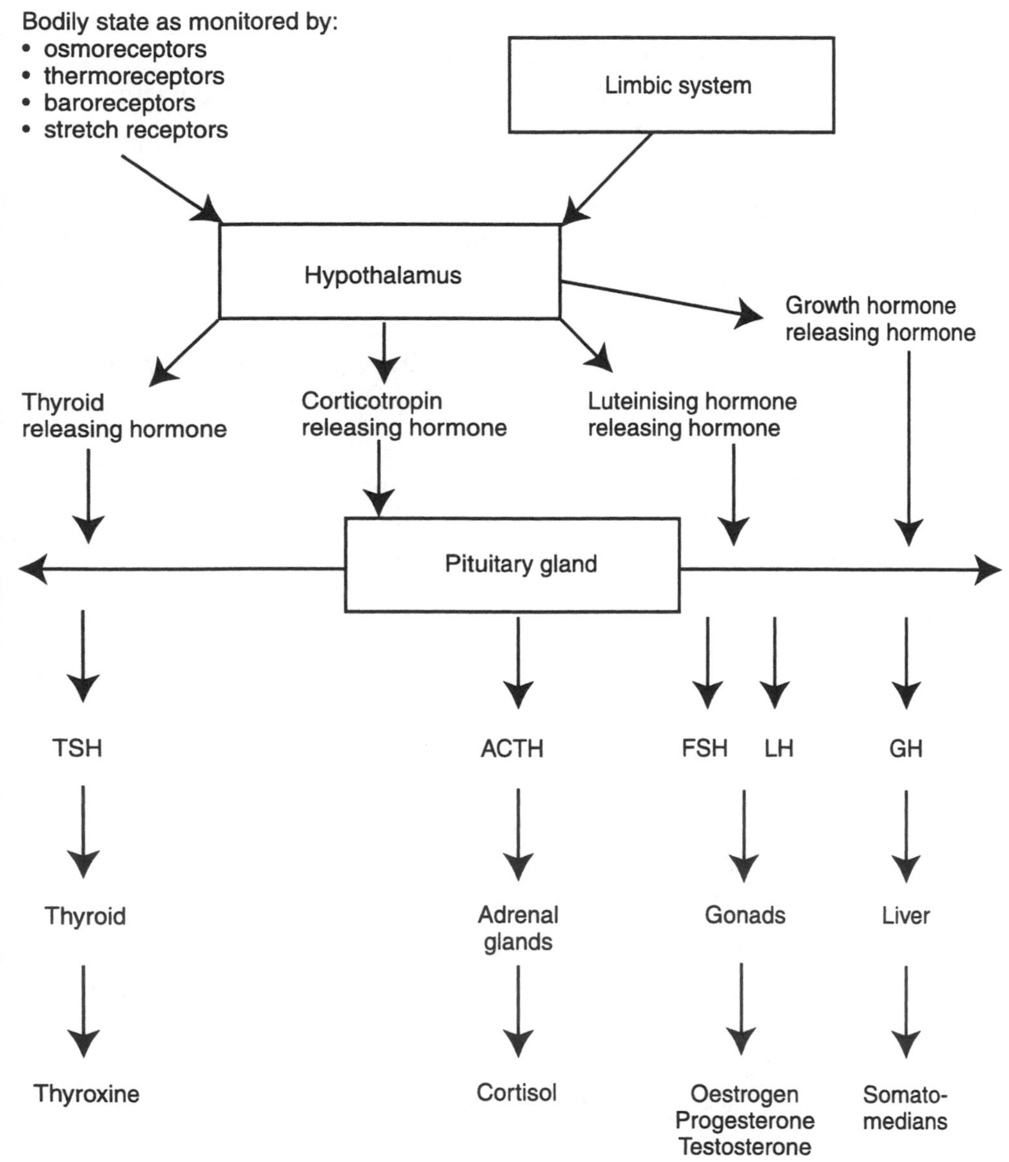

gure 10.3 The interrelationship of hypothalamic functions

rce: Adapted from Marieb and Hoehn 2007

Through neural connections, the hypothalamus stimulates a pituitary response to changes in the homeostatic feedback mechanisms, such as for energy requirements. For example, it will stimulate the thyroid gland to produce thyroxine into the blood when the child is cold. This will increase metabolic rate by stimulating the body cells to take up glucose and increase their activity and thus warm the blood and tissues. The neurons that regulate thyroid hormone release in the hypothalamus lie conveniently close to those that regulate appetite so the child will demand more food (calories) in cold weather.

The developing mind

Cognitive development

Cognitive development is what children can be perceived to do when they think, learn, remember, understand, judge and use ideas. Jean Piaget (1896–1980) studied the way all children learnt and the changes that occurred over time in the way they made sense of their world. He showed how children used schema, organising frameworks to their thinking, and how these changed as their brain matured and their experiences increased. He showed four stages of a spiral development: the sensori-motor, the pre-occupational, the concrete-operational and the formal-operational periods. Individual difference has been extensively researched through the concept of intelligence. Meadows (1996) proposes that intelligent children have good vocabularies, read well with comprehension, talk fluently and sensibly, make good decisions, plan well, apply knowledge to problems, determine how best to achieve goals and are interested in things around them.

In the developing nervous system, the nerve cells that constitute the brain and central nervous system develop patterns of connections and activity well before birth. They transmit substances that regulate nerve growth and differentiation and, by the time the foetus is eight weeks old, the lower part of the brain already has an elaborate structure. It is the subsequent timing and patterning of external stimuli which will then determine the precise detail of the eventual neural networks through the editing, sorting and pruning of connections. In the first six weeks after birth, the central nervous system neural network undergoes its greatest reduction to allow connections to be made that are precise and effective, but it is during the whole of childhood that these networks are refined with different parts of the brain maturing at different times in relation to experiences. Lateralisation of the brain occurs soon after conception; this is where particular functions appear located in one side of the brain or the other (Meadows 1996). The left side (hemisphere) of the brain deals with analytical thinking, logical processes and responds to information that is sequentially offered. The right hemisphere responds to more holistic information, is responsible for spatial perception, body image, artistic endeavour and processes information diffusely integrating by several inputs at any one time. Many left-handed children are good at drawing and practical work (the right side of the brain controls the left side of the body). Many girls enjoy social networks and story reading. However, there is debate as to the nature/nurture influence on stereotypes of female/male behaviour.

Personality

Children's genetic inheritance influences their personality type; it defines those enduring characteristics that are significant in interpersonal behaviour. Children all have common characteristics that make them human and are ones they have in common with their group norm such as gender, ethnic and cultural background, and intelligence. They also have individual traits that are formed from their particular family experiences and identify the way they deal with the world such as being happy-go-lucky, tentative or loving. As they grow up, they develop secondary traits which are less influential and less consistent, such as tastes, preferences and reactions to particular situations (Gross 2005).

Perception

Perception is not a passive process; it is not just a representation of the function of the senses although it depends on them. It is an active process of interpretation which is based on sensory information.

It is also a selective process, otherwise the child would be overcome by the constant input from eyes, ears, taste, touch and smell that bombards their conscious brain. It involves inference, and goes beyond what is seen and heard. It is organised; it relates what is sensed to a shape or pattern, defined as the 'set'. This 'set' is where the child will tend to perceive some preferred aspects of the available sense data and not others. It is individual to the child; it is complex and influenced by context, instruction, expectation, motivation, emotion, past experience, cultural factors and reward and punishment (Gross 2005). It has templates, such as the preference in the young baby for the face shape, and it relates what is sensed to the context in which the sense has been stimulated, such as the enjoyment of reading if cuddled up with a parent.

It is interesting to compare the perceptions of children with abnormal 'sets', such as those with a learning disability, those who are blind and those who are deaf. The blind child 'sees' things through touch and the deaf child 'hears' things through sight. It is interesting also to ask whether one can perceive one's world at different levels; for example, the children who takes a medication for attention deficit hyperactivity disorder (ADHD). These children receive a stimulant to their brain; some report a clearing of the 'fog' and their improved ability to concentrate on their day to day activities. Babies may be more perceptive than is thought, as they experience relatively more light sleep than older children. Adolescents may perceive many things at once on different levels when they do their homework, listen to music, stroke the cat on their lap and chew gum or it may be that they are receiving information from different modes and thus the thinking, hearing, touch and taste sensations do not block each other – in fact, they may enhance learning.

Other higher order functions have effect on perception such as motivation and emotion. Body needs, such as food, may be perceived as a threat to the anorexic child but a comfort to a baby. Rewards for good behaviour are used to modulate disturbed children's activities but these children may be difficult to handle when they are angry. Individual children may value particular activities such as football or pop music and role model themselves on those they perceive to be 'cool'. Quiet children will see the requirement to take part in the school play as stressful but would value the opportunity to watch animals on a visit to the zoo.

It is suggested that the earlier the ability is developed the more innate it may be. In the study of babies' vision, it has been identified that they can scan at forty-eight hours after birth, can accommodate to distance and have preference for complex shapes at two to four months. Psychologists such as Bowlby (1951), who studied attachment of infants in the first year of life, suggest this innate ability allows the young child to recognise a familiar face, learn who that person is and, in having regular repeated opportunities to look at that face, will develop strength and security within that bond. Vorria *et al.* (2006), in their study of 100 children's cognitive development at four years, showed how important this early attachment was. They found that when infants were cared for in institutions and then transferred to adoptive families they still scored lower in cognitive development than family reared children.

Memory

Memory is important to the learning process; it is important to make learning and experiences permanent in order to benefit from them. Without building up a network of memory, the world would present itself as a very dangerous place and survival would be short. There are three interrelated activities: reception of meaningful information, storage of this information and a method of retrieving it (Figure 10.4).

Sensory inputs, information on facts and skills, are processed by the cerebral cortex which selects about 5 per cent of the information to be stored. Many factors affect what facts and skills are remembered, such as emotion, repetition of information, association with the familiar and interesting 'other' information not related to the focus of attention. Children can be easily distracted by this 'other' information if they become bored with events or find them too difficult to comprehend. Sensory impulses are then channelled to the medial temporal lobe which includes the hippocampus and is part of the limbic area. The temporal area of the brain communicates with both the cortex (higher coordinating area) and the thalamus (lower coordinating centre), its neural pathways become established as changes occur in the nerve structures.

Marieb and Hoehn (2007) describes four changes that have been identified in nerve pathways involved in information storage and retrieval: new nucleic material is made in the nerve cell nuclei which allows the cell to undertake new functions; the cell membrane shape

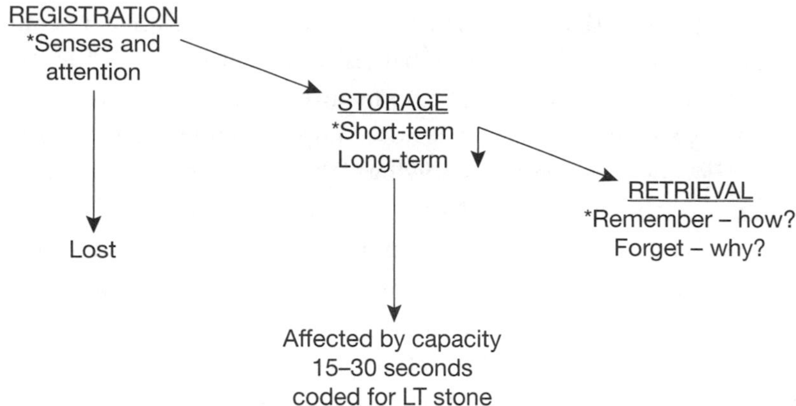

Figure 10.4 Memory circuit

changes to allow connections to other nerve cells to reform; new proteins are deposited between nerve cells to allow unique sharing of stimuli; and the number and size of the vesicles at the ends of the nerve axons enlarge to allow more chemicals to be secreted.

To understand why children forget, one must ask whether the information was stored in the first place or whether there is a block to retrieve the information. It appears that skills are less likely to be lost completely than facts. Children learn to swim and ride bicycles; they rarely lose skills once proficient. However, school homework facts seem to elude them regularly. Memory fades with time if: 1) it is displaced by other similar material; 2) it is not consolidated by repetition; 3) it does not have cues for retrieval; or 4) the child wants to forget, such as when they have had an unpleasant experience.

Motivation

Motivated behaviour is goal directed and purposeful. It is the 'drive' to survive and relates to both the physiological balance of the body systems and need to learn. The physiological is controlled by the hypothalamus and, as Maslow (1954) describes, these basic needs must be satisfied before 'higher order needs' of self actualisation can be addressed (see Figure 10.5). Children who are hungry and tired will not be curious to learn, they will not play or seek out satisfying activities that help them make sense of their world. Children who are frightened and live chaotic lives will have difficulty in becoming

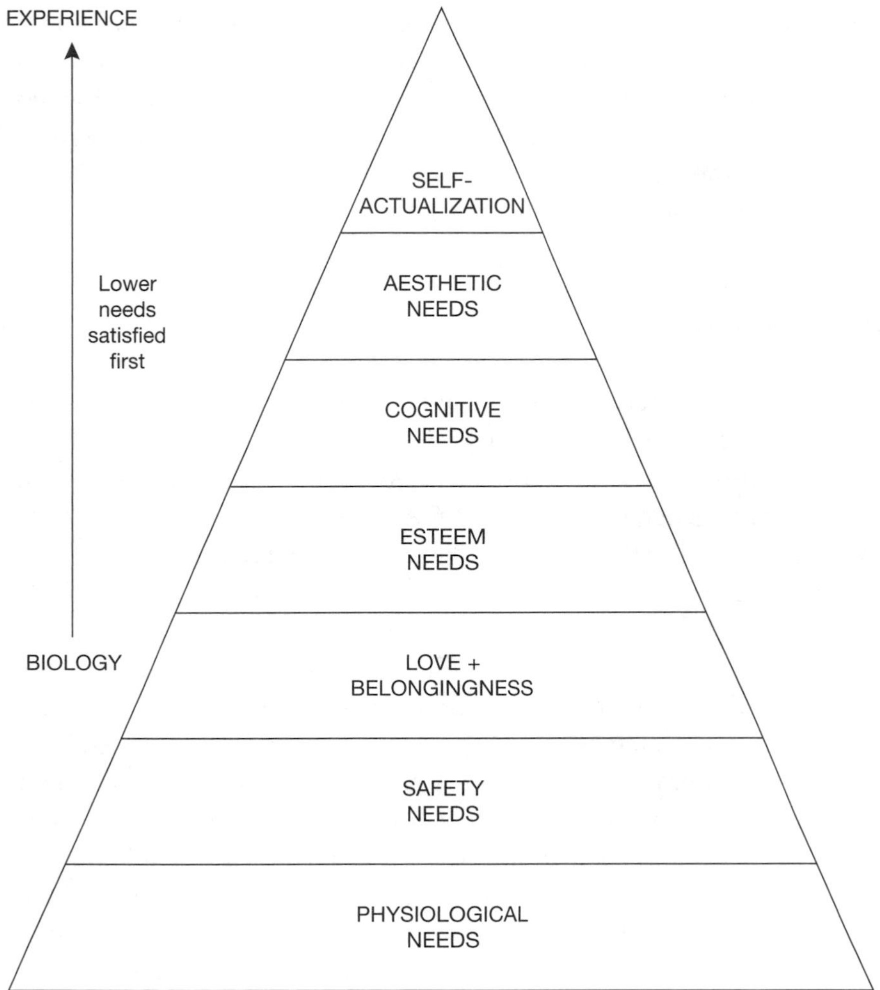

Figure 10.5 Maslow's hierarchy of needs

competent in social activity or appreciate the beauty and order within their own cultural environment.

Emotions are the subjective experiences related to physiological changes in the body. Happiness, sadness, pain and love are all words used to describe the phenomenon of emotion and are often measured by the individual child's report or subsequent behaviour. We infer that a child is happy when they smile and are relaxed, but some children can learn to produce the outward sign of something they do not feel to protect themselves from perceived danger. Pain can be measured by the physiological signs of stress, the raised heart rate and blood pressure, and the increased chemicals such as cortisol in the blood. Children can be distracted with favourite toys and video stories so they do not display pain behaviour and report they are 'OK', but their physiology will show that damaging chemicals are circulating through their body tissues.

Social development

Social cognition starts when the child recognises individuals (perceives) and uses facial expressions and gestures to communicate with them. Attachment (also an emotional development) is the first social relationship; general cognitive abilities are, here, used more specifically with people rather than objects. The development of social skills shows a changing quality as children mature. They change their attention from outer to inner characteristics. The young child will observe people talking together but an older child will try to find out what they are talking about and what they think about the topic. A young child will understand relationships through their immediate feelings, such as happiness or fear, whereas the older child will think about how the relationship should be; 'I love my Mum and I like to live with her' becomes ' I love my Mum and Dad so why can't we live with Mum and Dad as a family?'. Young children see their social world as constrained by social norms, such as 'Mum does the cooking'. The older child will see that Dad does the cooking when Mum is at work and Mum fills the car with petrol when she is using the car. Finally, children become less egocentric with time and eventually can see the world from another's point of view (Bee and Boyd 2007).

Socially adept children have learnt to read the cues in other's behaviour; this is a big challenge for the five-year-old starting school where teachers do not always consider their every, immediate, individual need and other children do not behave like the inanimate dolls of the bedroom when they play. Empathy also develops as children learn to read the emotional cues of others, such as being sad or angry. Individual temperament, family expectations and cultural influences are all influential in developing the skills to live and work in a group. Dosani (2006) reports on a conduct disorder prevention programme for parents, which was offered to 100 families in deprived districts of Jamaica. Parents were guided in active listening, child focused play, praise, limit setting, how to offer incentives for good behaviour and discipline methods to help children develop self control. This preventive programme aimed to help effective parenting was seen as a powerful protective factor which mitigated against socio-economic adversity. These identified deprived groups were suffering the consequences of 'out of control' adolescent gangs.

Moral development

Gross (2005) explains how moral development is the acquisition of rules that govern behaviour in a social world. It entails knowing what is right and wrong (cognitive), living within moral rules (behavioural) and having the ability to feeling shame, guilt or pride (emotional). He presents three famous psychologists who wrote on moral development: Freud who described the development of a conscience as a super-ego (the ideal person), a part of personality development; Piaget who described the understanding of moral standards within a child's general understanding of the world; and Kohlberg who designed moral dilemmas for children to solve and showed how moral development relies on but lags behind cognitive development. Kohlberg proposed nine universal moral values:

- punishment
- property
- law
- roles and concerns of affection and authority
- life
- liberty
- distributive justice
- truth
- sex.

However, although Gross accepts a developmental progression of understanding the world throughout childhood, he suggests that most of our moral responses are intuitive (emotional), that social rules are different to moral rules and that moral behaviour is often situational.

Children might know the 'right way' to behave but may choose another way when the peer group pressure affects them or when they see a short-term gain that is important for them at the time. Children might know to say sorry if they hurt another child but one could ask whether they actually feel (affective) sorry if they have, in fact, settled a long-standing 'score'. Societies have long produced shared myths and stories to teach history, cultural norms, and social and moral behaviour to their young. Many favourite children's stories persist, such as the story of Pinocchio, which explains moral behaviour in an amusing way. Pinocchio suffers the consequences of telling lies and eventually sees the benefit of selfless action with the help of his 'conscience', Jiminy Cricket. Many stories have been converted to film which show children the benefits of behaving in 'the right' way, such as Cinderella who wins her prince from the ugly sisters. Sadly, many role models and real life stories show children how lies and cruelty succeed; material wealth is often seen as the ultimate goal of a successful life rather than being an active member of a caring, sharing society.

Physiology knowledge in practice

Scenario 1

Peter, aged four years, wants to learn to ride a bike. What are the learning processes involved?

Some pointers:

- The first learning process is motivation. Motivation is strongest if the goal is focused. Peter wants to ride a bike which is his motivation towards the goal to ride the bike. There are other drivers towards his goal; the role model of the older children who ride bikes; his friends who can ride a bike and get enjoyment from it; his need for active physical play on exciting apparatus; the attention he will get from an adult who helps him acquire a new skill and the future hope of riding his bike away from his mother!
- Peter has to develop physical strength and fine coordination. This will depend on his nervous system maturing and his muscles being exercised in the activity he undertakes. Bike riding requires balance, leg muscle strength and skeletal flexibility.
- We assume Peter is within the normal range of intelligence and can understand his world. He would have experienced falls and being hurt so we would expect him to be apprehensive in his new venture.

- In learning a new skill, Peter aged 4 years, will be in Piaget's concrete operational skill development phase. This requires the learner to be shown a skill, be helped to practice it and become competent. When he is competent he will then start to transfer his skill to other activities such as riding his bike in more challenging circumstances. Look at small children and how they always try to do more.
- Peter will need to practice his new skill by repeating the activity. He will then store the experience in his memory. This will allow him to repeat bike riding at a later date and not have to return to the first principles of the activity.
- In achieving competence at bike riding Peter will feel a sense of achievement, which will make him feel good. Children often have a false sense of competence when they transfer a new skill and do not understand potential danger. Peter is only 4 years old, therefore his carers will have to anticipate danger for him at this age.

Scenario 2

Sally-Ann is fifteen years old and her teachers have noticed she is becoming thin and withdrawn at school. What are the 'drivers' for eating and what may Sally-Ann be feeling?

The theory

- As Sally-Ann's blood sugars fall, her body will not have glucose available for energy so she will feel tired, lethargic and irritable. Her body will try to compensate by releasing glucagon from the pancreas, which is a hormone that converts glycogen in the liver and muscles to glucose for release into the blood circulation.
- Sally-Ann's breath will begin to smell of pear drops and her mouth will feel dry. The liver makes acetone as it converts fats to glucose from the adipose stores of the body. This makes the blood acid. Acidity in the blood stimulates the respiratory centre in the brain to alter her breathing pattern. Acetone is excreted in the body fluids and exhaled from the lungs so expiration of air from the lungs will carry this chemical.
- Sally-Ann's abnormal behaviour is to acknowledge the feeling of hunger (the internal cue) and disallow it. She will respond to external cues which may be that she perceives herself to be too fat or avoidance of specific food that she fears will make her fat.

She may be 'punishing' herself for something of which she may not be totally aware such as family/peer group disruption.

- Sally-Ann's brain will respond to the lower blood sugars and her 'hunger centre' would normally drive her to seek food. Her increased peristalsis ('stomach rumbles') results from the hormone stimulus of the gut to prepare for food intake.
- She may eat because she has to; her social development allows her to respond to her parents instructions to eat with the family and her intellect tells her that if she conforms she will be released from the challenge of food. However, she may still vomit the food after the meal to control her gut absorbing the nutrients, and hide this behaviour from her family.

Extend your knowledge

Evans (2006), in his paper 'Child development and the physical environment', offers a range of physical environments that are detrimental to children's development. One of the topics he investigates is overcrowding and he reviews the effects on interpersonal relationships, mental health such as stress, motivation, and cognitive function. Think of how an overcrowded environment affects you; read Evans's article and discuss how parents can reduce the problems for their children in their local situation.

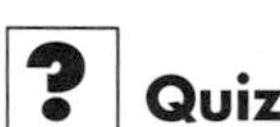

Quiz

Enter the words across to complete the matrix below.

1 Structure in the limbic area that responds to frightening experiences

2 We infer brain activity by watching children's _______

3 The cerebral cortex is responsible for this activity

4 The limbic area is the _______ brain

5 _______ cognition is about children's interactions with other people and their relationships with them

6 The structure in the limbic area that transfers experiences into memory

1							**G**									
2							**E**									
3							**N**									
4							**E**									
5							**S**									
6							**A**									
7							**N**									
8							**D**									
9							**E**									
10							**N**									
11							**V**									
12							**I**									
13							**R**									
14							**O**									
15							**N**									
16							**M**									
17							**E**									
18							**N**									
19							**T**									

7 One needs to attract the ______ of children to help them to do things

8 A child with an attention deficit may have this condition

9 To be aware through the senses

10 The development stage at which a child first fixes their vision on objects

11 An incentive or drive

12 The emotional brain

13 Development that allows children to distinguish right from wrong

14 The unconscious control centre of body functions

15 Development by which knowledge is acquired
16 Ability to retain information
17 The child's first attachment
18 Racial group influence on development
19 A shared social identity

Further reading

www.psycheducation.org/emotion/R%20complex.htm

Appendix

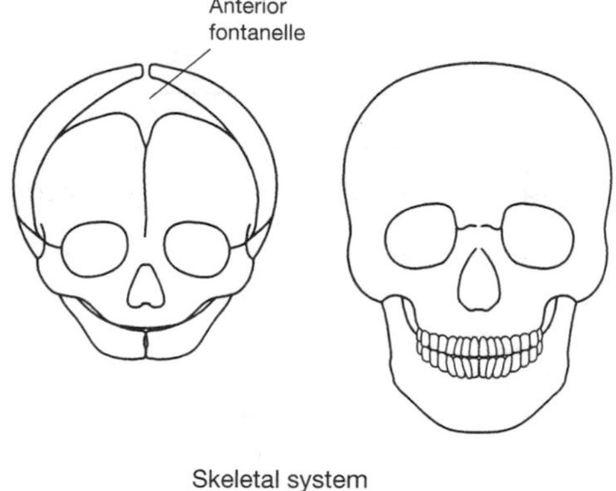

Figure 2.3 Bone structure in the infant and adolescent skull

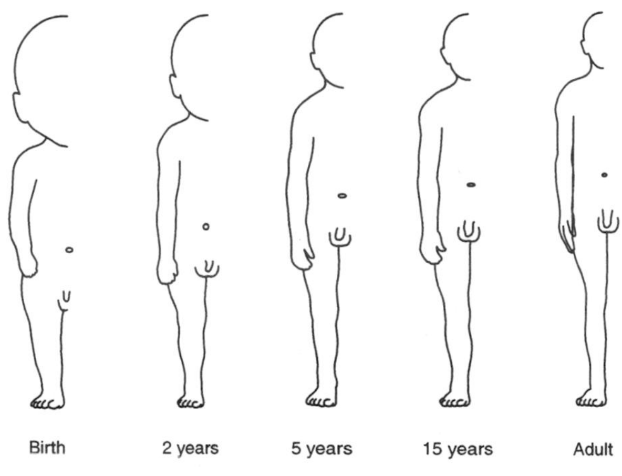

Figure 2.5 How body proportions change with age

Table 4.4 Heart rates in childhood

Age	*Rate*
Under 1 year	110–160
2–5 years	95–140
5–12 years	80–120
Over 12 years	60–100

Source: Lissauer and Clayden 2004

Table 4.5 Blood pressure changes over childhood

Age	*Male*	*Female*
1 year	80/34–89/39	83/38–90/42
5 years	90/50–98/55	89/52–96/56
10 years	97/58–106/63	98/59–105/62
15 years	109/61–117/66	107/64–113/67

Note: Reference adapted from American Academy of Pediatrics 2006 – values given reflect the fifth to ninety-fifth centile range of height in mm-Hg at rest.

Table 5.1 Respiratory rates in children

Age	*Rate*	*Too high*
Newborn	30–50	Over 60
1 year	26–40	Over 50
2 years	20–30	
4 years	20–26	Over 40
5 years	19–25	
6 years	18–24	
7 years	17–24	
8 years	17–23	
9 years	16–23	
10 years	15–22	
11 years	14–21	
12 years	14–21	
13 years	13–20	

Table 5.1 Respiratory rates in children *continued*

Age	*Rate*	*Too high*
14 years	12–20	
15 years	12–19	
16 years	11–14	

Source: Adapted from Wallis *et al.* (2005) for children at rest in the 2.5–97.5 centile range.

Note: Rates may be higher by 10 per cent if the child is awake, anxious or restless (Aylott 2006).

Table 6.1 Daily average fluid requirements for children calculated by body weight

Age	*Body weight in kg*	*Water (ml/kg/24 hours)*
Newborn	3	80–100
1 year	9.5	120–135
4 years	16.2	100–110
10 years	28.7	70–85
14 years	45	50–60

Table 6.2 Normal venous blood electrolyte values

Component	*Amount (mmols/l)*
Sodium	135–145
Potassium	3.5–4.5
Urea	2.5–4.5
Phosphate	0.8–1.4
Creatinine	0–6

Source: Glasper *et al.* 2007

Glossary

atheroma Deposition of lipids and other substances in the intima (inner layer) of the medium and large arteries. This then becomes thickened. Smooth muscle cells, collagen and elastic fibres accumulate and lipids, especially cholesterol, deposit on the artery wall, narrowing its lumen.

bifurcation To fork or lead into two pathways.

chondroitin sulphate The organic matrix of bone imparts its tensile strength. Of this matrix, 95 per cent is collagen with hyaluronic acid and chondroitin sulphate constituting 5 per cent. The mineral matrix consists of amorphous calcium phosphate and a crystalline structure such as hydroxy-apatite.

cytoplasm Cellular substance between the plasma membrane and the nuclear membrane. It typically contains proteins, organic polyphosphates, nucleic acids and other ionised substances that cannot permeate the plasma membrane. The majority of these impermeant intracellular ions are negatively charged at physiological pH.

dendrites Neuron cytoplasm processes which increase the surface area of the nerve cell body to be available for connections to other nerve bodies.

desquamated epithelium The shed lining (epithelium) of the gut.

gemoglossus muscle A triangular muscle attached by a short tendon to the inner surface of the mandible symphysis. It spreads out in a fan-like form to attach to the hyoid bone, muscles of the pharynx and the whole length of the under surface of the tongue. This muscle draws the tongue forward and protrudes the apex through the mouth. It draws the middle of the tongue down to make the upper surface concave from side to side.

glomerular filtration The process where fluid from the blood is forced under pressure out of tiny capillaries (the glomerulus) in the kidney into tiny tubes (the nephron) where reabsorption of substances useful to the body such as sugar are reabsorbed and waste products such as urea are carried out of the kidney to the ureter and bladder for excretion.

human genome The human genome is the chemical structure of all forty-six chromosomes in a human cell nucleus.

hyperpyrexia (or fever) This is when the body temperature rises to a level where cell metabolism is disrupted. Many centres would consider 39 °C as a measurement at which to initiate antipyretic medication.

hypothalamus (or 'master gland') A small area of brain tissue deep inside the skull.

intermediate mesoderm A layer of cells between the endoderm and ectoderm which differentiates in the first stage of embryo development. It develops into the connective tissues, teeth, muscles, circulatory and lymph systems, urogenital tract and the endothelial linings of the pericardial, pleural and peritoneal cavities.

kernicterus This is caused by damage to cells in the basal ganglia of the brain due to excessive accumulation of bilirubin in the blood plasma after birth. The child develops motor difficulties in all parts of the body. It is seen when the child tries to initiate movement under voluntary control. Limbs jerk, facial expressions distort and speech is irregular.

lipoprotein Transport of non-polar lipids (fats) in plasma requires that they are joined with a protein. This occurs in the liver. The protein part of the lipoprotein then serves catalytic functions and interacts with specific cell receptors to facilitate endocytosis of fat into the cells.

metabolic alkalosis This is when the body fluids' pH rises above neutral (pH 7.45) and becomes alkaline. The bicarbonate ions in the blood increase. It is different to respiratory alkalosis where blood carbon dioxide (which is relative to its acidity) is reduced. This occurs in conditions of overbreathing where carbon dioxide from the lungs is lost in excess of inhalation of oxygen.

mitochondria Small organelles in the cell cytoplasm. They are the site of aerobic cellular respiration. ATP (adenosine triphosphate) is produced in them which stores energy released from the breakdown of glucose. This is called oxidative phosphorylation.

myelination This is where certain neuroglia surround neuron processes called axons and form a fatty sheath which insulates it and speeds up nerve impulses. In children this process takes many years to complete and thus control of movement, for example, matures with age.

osmolality The number of osmoles per kilogram of solvent. An osmole is a solution's ability to induce osmosis, thus it is a measurement of osmotic pressure.

parasympathetic reflexes These nervous stimuli are initiated by the hypothalamus and result in effects of relaxation, food processing and energy absorption. The effects are usually brief and are restricted to specific organs and sites.

phagocytes Leucocytes, usually neutrophils and monocytes. They engulf and destroy antigenantibody complexes, bacteria, protozoa, dead cells and foreign matter.

stratum germinativum At the epiphyscal growth plate, cartilage cells known as chondrocytes are arranged in columns extending from the epiphysis towards the shaft. The outer zone furthest from the shaft is where chondrocytes are more actively dividing. This is called the stratum gernunativum.

stratum spinosum This layer of developing bone takes its name from the process of ossification where chondrocytes hypertrophy and the lacunae around them expand to form irregular cavities in the matrix called spiculcs.

transient bradicardia A short period of slow heartbeat often brought about by stimulation of the vagus nerve in the neck during intuhation or passing a naso-gastric tube.

Answers to quizzes

1 Child physical needs

1. Be healthy. Stay safe. Enjoy and achieve. Make a positive contribution. Achieve economic wellbeing.
2. Material wellbeing, family and peer relationships, health and safety, behaviour and risks, educational wellbeing and subjective wellbeing.
3. The way in which children are the same and different; the internal and external influences on these changes; whether changes are quantitative or qualitative in nature.
4. There is a high correlation for a child and their parent regarding height, weight, shape and form of features, body build and skin colour. Many dimensions of personality, such as temperament, also seem to be inherited.
5. Stress from lack of appropriate food, love and safety.
6. Children are seen as adventurous, unpredictable and fun-seeking.
7. Children of this age group have a need to establish themselves as independent and responsible for their own actions, and this command over their own lives may lead them to feel indestructible.
8. Behavioural expressions, such as the frozen watchfulness in the toddler, overfriendliness in the school-aged child and the teenager who looks for a confidante, groomed by an abuser, should alert the professional carer to a child needing protection.
9. A secure attachment is needed to attain his or her full intellectual potential, sort out what he or she perceives, think logically, develop a conscience, become self-reliant, cope with stress and frustration, handle fear and worry, develop future relationships, handle jealousy.
10. Healthy social cognitive development stages move from outer to inner characteristics where a young child pays attention to the surface of

things, what things look like; the older child looks for principles, for causes. From observation to inference: the young child bases its conclusions on what they can see or feel; the older child will make inferences about what ought to be or might be. From definite to qualified: the young child's rules are fixed whereas the older child will 'bend' the rules to suit different contexts. From an observer's view to general rule: the child becomes less egocentric and is able to use experience to construct a view more applicable to everyone.

11 The schedule at present offers protection against diphtheria, tetanus, pertussus, polio haemophilus (DTaP/IPV/Hib) and pneumococcus at two months, DTaP/IPV/Hib with meningitis C (MenC) at three months, DTaP/IPV/Hib with pneumococcus protection at four months, Hib and MenC at twelve months, measles, mumps and rubella with pneumococcus at thirteen months, boosters for MMR/DTaP/IPV vaccinations at three to five years and boosters for dT/IPV at thirteen to eighteen years.

12 In the prevention of cervical cancer initiative, where ten-year-old girls can be offered a five-year protection from incubating the papillomavirus – a viral infection transmitted during sexual intercourse – parents are unhappy with the sexual health knowledge needed to advise this age group.

13 At birth the baby can depend on colostrum, a thin, yellowish fluid which is particularly valuable for the establishment of lactobacilli in the gut, and contains less fat and energy but more secretory IgA immunoglobulin than later breast milk. Mature breast milk, produced at ten to fourteen days after birth, is unique in that its composition varies over the course of a feed, a day and the period of lactation. Lactose is the principal carbohydrate of mature breast milk, providing about 39 per cent of the energy for the baby. Proteins composing 60 per cent whey to 40 per cent casein are particularly easily digested, and predominantly long-chain fatty acids provide 50 per cent of all energy requirements until the age of four months, when the gut physiology is matured and weaning to solids can commence. Breast milk also contains a number of anti-infective properties such as macrophages, IgA, lysozyme, lactoferrin, interferon and bifidus factor, which appear to protect the infant from respiratory and gastrointestinal infections in the first six months of life.

14 A healthy diet should be based on a wide variety of foods, with emphasis on those foods of high nutrient density rather than those providing energy only, for children under five years. This balanced diet can be achieved by selecting items from four food groups each day: three can be taken from lean meat, fish, poultry, game, eggs, pulses and nuts; three from milk, cheese and yoghurt; four from bread, rice, pasta, breakfast cereal and potatoes; and four from vegetables and fruit.

15 Vegetarianism, teenage pregnancy, sports and athletic training, smoking, drinking alcohol and sliming diets have profound effect on long-term health for this age group. The adolescent, however, lives in the 'immediate' world and healthy eating behaviour may not fit with their daily routines and peer group pressure.
16 Poor eating habits, lack of exercise, emotional need, rarely genetic abnormality but must be alert for Pader Willi Syndrome.
17 Can not move to get warm, large surface area to body mass ratio thus loses heat to environment, large head to trunk ratio, reduced subcutaneous fat to insulate body, may be unwell and not feeding – thus reduced calorie intake.
18 Day out in the woods/parks, to the seaside, sports centre for activities such as cycling, tennis and swimming, and interest centres such as castles and historic sites where there is room to run and relax.
19 Fitness in children can be measured by their cardiovascular endurance, blood pressure, blood lipid profile, fatness and glucose tolerance – their metabolic fitness.
20 All children need to sleep, it is then that they grow and repair of body tissues occurs.

2 The skeletal system

1 Two groups of bone cells work antagonistically through life to maintain the skeleton. Osteoblasts are modified fibroblasts which have collagen fibres deposited round them; calcium salts then accumulate here to increase bone size. Osteoclasts, developed from the bone marrow stem cells, then continually shape bone by removing excess material.
2 Ossification of many bones occurs in the second month of foetal life. The clavicle and bones of the skull vault ossify 'in membrane' as blood vessels penetrate the area and bring in osteoblasts and osteoclasts. Other bones ossify as the connective tissue converts to a cartilage template and then to bone. These starting points for bone ossification are called primary centres, and appear in different bones at different times.
3 The vertebral spine has two primary curves present at birth, but normally by adolescence four vertebral curves are evident; the cervical (lordotic), the thoracic (primary curve), the lumbar (lordotic) and the sacral (primary curve).
4 The jaw is small at birth with usually no teeth, but grows until puberty when adult proportions are apparent. Resuscitation in children under seven years of age demands a different technique to that of adults, as the head and neck anatomy results in relatively high positions of larynx and trachea and the rib cage is more compliant.

5 Growth is influenced by normal inheritance, physiological age, normal variation in nutritional status, health, hormonal status and antenatal history.
6 Parents will report periods of rapid growth and periods of little change in height – the 'Christmas tree pattern'.
7 Somatomedian is secreted by the proliferative cells in the growth plate as well as the liver, which is the main source of this hormone.
8 Local growth is controlled by chalones which are chemicals that balance the cell division and differentiation phases in tissue growth; they are formed by actively dividing cells. They are also secreted by cells adjacent to dividing cells in their cell membranes to control cell spacing. Age of tissue, and its mitotic ability, influence chalone secretion, thus the growing child replaces damaged tissue quickly after injury.
9 It stimulates the uptake of amino acids from the blood and their incorporation into proteins and the reduction of protein breakdown for cellular energy release; stimulates the uptake of the mineral sulphur needed for the synthesis of chondroitin sulphate into the cartilage matrix; stimulates the mobilisation of fats from adipose tissue for transport to cells, thus increasing the blood levels of fatty acids for cell uptake and energy release; reduces glucose uptake by cells for energy release, thus increases blood glucose levels.
10 It acts on the skeleton by inhibiting bone reabsorption and the release of ionic calcium from the bony matrix. It stimulates calcium uptake from the blood and its incorporation into the bone matrix by the osteoblasts. It increases the excretion of calcium and phosphate ions by the kidney. Raised blood calcium (over 20 per cent) stimulates its release.
11 Stressed children do not grow as they have a chronic raised metabolic rate. Cortisol also converts non-carbohydrates, that is fats and proteins, to glucose for energy, thus reducing the availability of these nutrients for tissue development. High levels of glucocorticoids depress cartilage and bone formation and reduce muscle mass. Chronically stressed children will use all their nutrients for energy release rather than for tissue building.
12 In females they contribute to the development of libido and are converted to oestrogen by body tissues. They sustain the growth of axilla and pubic hair at puberty and contribute to the development of 'teenage spots' in males and females.
13 The production of insulin is halted by somatostatin, which is secreted by both the hypothalamus, the pancreas D cells and throughout the gastrointestinal tract. The major effect of somatostatin is to inhibit insulin and glucagon local to the pancreas where most of it is secreted. It also inhibits digestive function by reducing gut motility, gastric secretion and pancreatic endocrine function and absorption at the gut mucosa, thus, paces foodstuff conversion.

14 Oestrogen also has an anabolic effect in puberty, particularly on the female reproductive system. The breasts grow, subcutaneous fat increases, the pelvis widens and calcium is facilitated into the skeleton. Oestrogen also supports her skeletal growth spurt until high enough levels are reached to close the epiphyseal plates and stop long bone growth and, thus, height. Low oestrogen levels have been found to have a powerful effect in offsetting the positive bone mass accumulation promoted by calcium in the diet and by weight bearing exercise.

15 Testosterone levels rise at puberty in males when this hormone effect leads to the increase in bone growth and density and skeletal muscle size and mass. Testosterone boosts the basic metabolic rate at all stages of the male child's life.

16 The proportion of calcium uptake compared to body weight is highest in the term foetus, where 300 mg calcium passes through the placenta each day, as compared with the teenager, who requires 800–1000 mg.

17 Physical activity of three hours per week, which starts before the pre-pubertal growth spurt, in activities such as gymnastics, football/handball increases the lean mass of skeletal muscle. This tissue will give maximum tension on developing bones to ensure optimal mineral mass accrual.

18 Muscle structure is determined at birth by the genetic inheritance. As muscles mature their ability to contract is more efficient. Together with their growth in size, so strength increases.

19 In the adolescent spurt the feet and hands grow first, then the calf and forearm, hips and chest, then the shoulders. Adolescent children are often accused of being clumsy; however, their bodies may have grown at such a rate that their brains have not yet reorganised spatially.

20 Toddlers who can jump in puddles will experience mastery over their world; eight-year-olds who can ride a bike will experience the thrill of attaining a skill; the young person who sees an adult body emerging will need to constantly reshape his or her identity. Physical change will also determine new social roles and expectations, and children who are too small or too big compared to their peer group will experience advantages and disadvantages in equal measure.

3 The nervous system

1 The first indication of the nervous system is the neural plate, a thickened area of the ectoderm. It is induced to form early in the third week, and by the end of this week the neural folds have begun to fuse to the median plane to form the neural tube. This neural tube is the beginning of the brain and spinal cord. As the neural tube separates from the surface ectoderm cells, the neural folds form the neural crest. Ganglia of the spine, cranial and autonomic nervous system develop from the neural crest.

2 The two hemispheres of the human brain are not mirror images of each other; the upper surface of the temporal lobe and the whole occipital region is larger on the left side than on the right. The perception functions of the left brain are more specialised for the analysis of stimuli sequences which occur one after the other whereas the right brain analyses space, shape and form which are presented at the same time. The right hemisphere processes spatial information, both visual and tactile.
3 The first part of the cortex to develop is the primary motor area located in the pre-central gyrus, the cells which initiate movement. The second area to develop is the primary sensory area in the post-central gyrus where nerve fibres mediate the sense of touch. The third area to develop is the primary visual area in the occipital lobe where nerve paths from the retina end.
4 The anterior fontanelle, which can be felt in the midline of the skull above the brow, closes gradually in the first eighteen months of life, while the smaller posterior fontanelle, again in the midline but towards the back of the baby's head, is normally closed by the age of six weeks.
5 Heat is created by metabolism in the liver, skeletal muscles and other chemical actions. Metabolism releases chemical energy from the covalent bonds of hydrogen compounds, fat and carbohydrates, and the energy that is not used for cell activity is lost as heat. Also shivering, which is the involuntary and spasmodic contraction and relaxation of skeletal muscles, creates heat by muscle work. The pilomotor reflex, which makes hair on the skin stand up due to contraction of the pilomotor muscles in the hair follicles, traps air near the skin surface and insulates it from loss of body heat through convection. Parents and carers may observe changes in skin colour, posture, fluid intake and output, and level of activity and behaviour.
6 Oligodendrocytes are responsible for myelination of axons in the central nervous system. They can myelinate several processes at any one time. Schwann cells ensheath the axons of peripheral nerve axons. Their myeline sheath of 80 per cent lipids and 20 per cent protein insulates the nerve axon and allows rapid transmission of nerve impulse. Myelination of the nerve axons is a process that continues after birth. The nodes of Ranvier, spaces between the Schwann cells, appear constant as the nerve axon grows. As the internodal spaces elongate, the speed of transmission of the nerve impulse increases. In general, the thicker the nerve the thicker the myeline sheath that wraps around it. Satellite cells encapsulate dorsal root and cranial nerve ganglion cells and regulate their micro-environment. Astrocytes occupy interneurone spaces and connect to small blood vessels, thus allowing neurone nutrition. Their processes surround groups of synaptic endings in the central nervous

system and isolate them from adjacent synapses. Their foot processes connect the blood vessels with the connective tissue at the surface of the central nervous system, which may help limit the free diffusion of substances into the central nervous system itself. Microglia transform to phagocyte when cells in the nervous system are damaged, and are probably derived from the circulation. Ependymal cells line the ventricles of the brain and separate the chambers for the central nervous system tissue. Many substances diffuse easily across them between the extracellular space of the brain and the cerebral spinal fluid.

7 The blood/brain barrier is an anatomical/physiological feature of the brain that separates brain parenchyma from blood. It is formed chiefly by tight junctions between capillary endothelial cells of the blood vessels. These cerebral capillaries have no fenestrations or pores, and are thought to be responsible for the selective nature of the blood/brain barrier when mature. The blood/brain barrier is a term used to describe its function, based on observations that facilitated diffusion of glucose. Essential amino acids, some electrolytes and passive diffusion of water and carbon dioxide is allowed, but it is impermeable to non essential amino acids and potassium ions.

8 The blood/brain barrier functions to exclude substances that are of low solubility in lipid, such as organic acids, highly ionised polar compounds, large molecules and substances not transported by specific carrier-mediated transport systems. These include albumin and substances bound to albumin such as bilirubin, many hormones and drugs, organic and inorganic toxins.

9 Blink, the corneal and blinking reflexes are strong and can be seen when the baby is carried in a draught or faced towards the sun. Yawn, cough, sneeze, defecate and micturate, taste and smell and withdraw from pain. Cry, root, suck, swallow – these primitive reflexes associated with feeding, the tongue retrusion reflex, are well developed at birth. Grasp a finger if placed in the palm of the hand, this palmer grasp is a flexor response and is characterised by a relatively strong flexion of the palm and fingers without thumb opposition and will curl the foot if the plantar surface is equally stroked (Babinski sign). Show a startle reflex (Moro sign) if his/her position is quickly changed. The Moro reflex, where the startled child will fling his or her arms symmetrically apart and then bring them together again, is the most consistent primitive developmental milestone between birth and three months. The extensor response can be demonstrated by any sudden movement of the neck region. The infant reacts with extension and abduction of the extremities and a noticeable tremor of the hands and feet. Show the startle reflex, which is similar to the Moro and is stimulated by a loud unexpected noise; the baby responds as to the Moro response but with flexion rather than abduction of the extremities.

10 One of these is the tonic neck reflex. This develops in the first few months of life. When the baby's head is turned to one side he or she responds with an increased muscle tone and extension of both the arm and the leg of the side to which the face is turned, and by the flexion of the arm and leg of the opposite side. Another postural reflex, the righting reflex, facilitates maintenance of the relationship between the head and other body parts. The third postural reflex, the labyrinthine reflex, orientates the body relative to the force of gravity. These postural reflexes begin to emerge at about three months and increase in intensity throughout infancy. Their function is to help the baby maintain or regain its balance against gravity when disturbed.

11 The tiny baby has acute skin sensation, but as the child grows the skin receptors become more differentially spaced, widely spaced particularly over the dorsal surface of the body but more concentrated in areas such as breast and inner thigh where skin remains more sensitive to touch.

12 Both boys and girls produce oil onto the skin, oil glands in the skin are activated by the androgens of the adrenal cortex; the control of overactive sebaceous glands and infections in acne causes difficulty for the emerging adult. Boys produce more sweat than girls because of the higher muscle mass and heat production, but both become better protected from the sun as melanin production achieves mature function.

13 Children need to focus light on to the central part of the retina, the fovea, for the colour receptors, cones, to develop. There seems to be a critical time for development of the fovea, about the age of three to four years.

14 Sound waves move air molecules, focused by the pinna to the external meatus, that impact on the tympanic membrane at the end of the passage from the outer ear. This membrane vibrates and moves the three bones of the middle ear which, in turn, vibrate against the inner ear membrane, a communication window to the fluid filled cochlea. In the cochlea the fluid waves disrupt fine hairs that stimulate the auditory nerve. The auditory nerve then transmits a nerve impulse to the temporal lobe for interpretation by the cerebral cortex of the brain.

15 At four to seven months the production of more sophisticated sound increases in vocal play where the child gains control of articulation of the larynx and mouth and experiments in loudness, pitch and the position of the tongue. Children of this age love to play games that require them to practise this skill, sometimes inappropriately at meal times.

16 The control of movement improves as the myeline increases and the child interacts with the environment. Although there is a wide range of normal movements, the sequence of development shows the same steps. First is the cephalocaudal, or head-to-toe development, as the child shows the ability to control the head and face before the lower limbs.

17 Motor development is a plastic process, and variation in the sequence, timing and rate of development is most likely to relate to a variety of biological (genetic, body size and composition) and environmental (rearing atmosphere, play opportunities and objects) factors.
18 Sleep is universal among higher vertebrates and is defined as a state of partial consciousness from which one can be roused by stimulation. This differentiates it from coma from which one cannot easily be woken.
19 Superimposed on this mechanism are circadian rhythms, which are thought to be controlled by the suprachiasmic nuclei situated near the third ventricle in the brain which connects the retina of the eye to the specialised nerve endings. Our body rhythms are also controlled by external clues, called zeitgebers, such as light, dark and daily temperature changes.
20 Sleep is induced by complex neuro-chemical reactions arising in the tissues of the brain stem known as the reticular formation and mediated by neurotransmitters such as serotonin and noradrenaline. Superimposed on this mechanism are circadian rhythms, which are thought to be controlled by the suprachiasmic nuclei situated near the third ventricle in the brain which connects the retina of the eye to the specialised nerve endings.

4 The cardiovascular system

1 In the fourth week after conception a pair of angioblastic cords develop from the mesoderm to form a pair of endocardial tubes, which then fuse to form the primitive heart tube.
2 In the foetal circulation oxygenated blood enters the body through the left umbilical vein.
3 The umbilical artery.
4 At birth this is at 18 g per dl.
5 The current recommendation in the UK is to commence weaning at six months and to supplement the feeds with iron before this time if the infant is bottle-fed on cow's milk. Breastfed babies can extract 50 per cent of their iron needs whereas bottle-fed babies can only extract 10 per cent from cow's milk. Thus, a substitute milk feed formula has iron added.
6 The average blood volume in the full-term infant is 85 ml per kg.
7 For red cell production the red marrow must have supplies of amino acids, iron, vitamins B12 and B6, and folic acid.
8 This is to test for phenylalanine found in 1:7,000–10,000 live births. It is an autosomal recessive disorder. Excess of this chemical shows that

the child's liver is not converting phenyalanine to tyrosine, an essential amino acid for tissue growth. Phenylketanuria (PKU) will lead to brain damage if undetected and not treated with an adjusted protein diet from birth. The child will usually be tested by heel prick on the sixth day of life after milk feeds have been established.

9 At birth, platelets are 150–450 × 10^9/l and remain stable for life.

10 The Apgar score taken at one minute and five minutes after birth is scored for a pulse which is either absent (zero points), or lower than 100 (1 point) or above 100 (2 points). These scores are added to scores from other critical measurements (linked to respiratory, muscular skeletal and nervous systems) and together they predict satisfactory survival of the infant.

11 Children of different sizes have different normal ranges of cardiac output, thus the cardiac index (CI) is often used for them: CI = CO divided by body surface in metres squared (normal is 3.5–4.5 l/min/m^2 of body surface).

12 A fall in systemic perfusion can be observed when the child becomes mottled and pale in colour; peripheral vasoconstriction occurs; peripheral extremities become cool; there is delayed capillary refill; decreased urine output is seen; and a metabolic acidosis is evident.

13 Heart rate measurements over childhood reflect a decreasing basic metabolic rate.

14 95–140.

15 Children's response to exercise is related to their age, the type of exercise undertaken and the gradual effect of physical activity in their day to day life.

16 Boys show an increasing haemoglobin concentration as they grow older when testosterone has an increasing effect on the growth spurt and development of secondary sexual characteristics in their late teens. Girls, on the other hand, show a lower increase in haemoglobin levels by menarche; thus teenage boys show superiority in endurance events because their blood is able to carry oxygen more efficiently to working muscles.

17 97/58–106/63.

18 Measurement of a child's blood pressure can be an inexact science as it becomes anxious when its arm or leg is compressed; the correct cuff bladder is also vital as systolic readings can be as much as 20 mmHg in error and hypertension erroneously diagnosed.

19 Social deprivation, family history of CVD, raised BMI (ratio of height to weight), high B/P outside the accepted range for age and smoking.

20 Weight control, regular exercise and a diet low in animal fats have been shown to reduce serum cholesterol.

5 The respiratory system

1 In the term infant there is a transition of breathing from episodic irregular, ineffectual movements to regular, rhythmic and effectual effort which is completed by the end of the first week of life.

2 Lungs appear as a bud from the oesophagus below the pharyngeal pouches at week five.

3 The lungs are filled with fluid so the alveoli are hypoxic and no gas exchange can take place (the mechanism for blood vessels round the lung to open and close is related to the availability of oxygen in the alveoli). This ensures that pulmonary vasoconstriction remains.

4 At twenty-two weeks' gestation surfactant is being secreted, with a surge in its production at thirty to thirty-five weeks and at birth.

5 Surfactant mixes with the water and loosens the cohesive tension at the film surface which reduces the pull to collapse the sacs and makes it easier for them to expand with air.

6 Mild cooling, light, sound, touch, odours and added gravity force, combined with the internal stimuli of reduced blood oxygen and rising carbon dioxide levels in the blood (increasing acidity), stimulate the respiratory centre in the brain and the infant should then take its first breath of air.

7 Infants up to four weeks are obligatory nose breathers, thus the risk to their breathing increases if they have colds or lie with their face in vomit or bedding.

8 At puberty, the larynx of a male will enlarge more than that of the female under the influence of rising testosterone levels in the blood, and the vocal cords will become thicker and stronger and thus produce the lower voice tones of the adult male.

9 When a small child makes respiratory effort the chest wall is more compliant (stretchy) than the adult, because only the external intercostal muscles, which elevate the ribs for inspiration, stabilise the chest wall. The diaphragm is more horizontal and there is lower rib retraction when the child lies supine. The greater the rib retraction the more the diaphragm will need to contract to generate tidal volume; this is a very inefficient way to breathe and the muscles will tire quickly when ventilation is increased for long periods.

10 This is a period of breathing absence lasting twenty seconds or more, or a shorter time if the child develops a bluish or pale colour or the heart rate drops.

11 Paediatric 'modifiers' to adult resuscitation procedure; give five initial breaths before starting chest compression; if on your own, perform one minute CPR (cardio-pulmonary resuscitation) before going for help;

compress the chest approximately one third of its depth. Use two fingers for an infant under one year; use one or two hands for a child over one year – they are needed to achieve an adequate depth of compression.

12 Respiratory rates tend to be slightly higher in boys, perhaps due to their changing lean body mass as they approach puberty and their increase in lean muscle tissue which has a higher metabolic demand for oxygen than fat.

13 Compliance is determined by the elastic properties of the lung, connective tissues and the alveolar surface forces, as well as the chest wall.

14 Twenty to twenty-six breaths per minute and over forty would be too high.

15 Peak expiratory flow (PEF) is a simple test of lung function; the highest flow achieved from a maximal forced expiratory manoeuvre started without hesitation from a position of maximal lung inflation.

16 Over long periods of aerobic activity they are disadvantaged because, although their oxygen uptake is at least as good as adults, they have smaller stores of muscle glycogen and immature temperature regulation systems.

17 Slowing of respiratory rate occurs as the child slips into the deep sleep state. The parasympathetic nerve supply dominates regulation of airway function; the bronchi/bronchiole muscles relax and reduce their lumen size.

18 In REM sleep, where dreaming occurs, respiration becomes irregular and the respiratory muscle activity is altered. Tonic intercostal muscle activity is partly abolished and rhythmic activity is reduced, phasic diaphragm activity compensates. There is a small decrease in ventilatory response to hypoxia, and loss of the tonic and inspiratory phase is also linked to relaxing of the throat muscles. Tidal volume, the amount of air moved in one inspiration, reduces.

19 In the upper respiratory tract, air enters the trachea via the nose and throat. The ear is closely connected to these passages by the Eustachian tube which is composed partly of bone and partly of cartilage and fibrous tissue and lined with mucosa. It extends from the middle ear to the nasopharynx (the part of the throat behind the nose) and allows equalisation of pressure either side of the tympanic membrane to avoid its rupture.

20 The anatomy of the young child's upper respiratory tract is small and structures are relatively close together, thus infections such as the common cold causing inflammation of the lining mucosa in the nasal passages and pharynx will soon involve other associated structures in the ear.

6 The renal system

1 Nephrons.
2 This is 70 per cent in the infant, decreasing over childhood to 60 per cent in the adult.
3 Water is mainly present in two 'compartments'; two thirds in the intracellular spaces and one third in the extra cellular spaces (80 per cent of this in the interstitial spaces and 20 per cent in the plasma). There are other pockets of fluid in many other parts of the body serving vital functions; this 'third compartment' consists of fluids such as the lymph fluid, cerebral spinal fluid, parts of the eye and ear, fluid in the pleural, pericardial and peritoneal cavities.
4 In the child there is a higher amount of the water outside the cells in the interstitial spaces, and a higher turnover of water due to an immature kidney function to conserve water. Young children also have a larger surface area × volume ratio and are therefore vulnerable to excess water loss from breathing and sweating to the outside environment. They have a larger circulating blood volume per kilogram of body weight, but their overall volume is small.
5 1,600–1,782 ml.
6 The kidney changes three times before it is completed.
7 Amniotic fluid is vital to the foetal development as it contains proteins, carbohydrates, lipids and phospholipids, urea and electrolytes. The amniotic fluid protects the foetus by cushioning it from outside crushing, allows it move and develop its muscular-skeletal system, keeps it at an even temperature and allows the lungs and gut to mature.
8 The neonate will pass 20–35 ml of urine four times a day while intake is low and milk production establishes in the mother, but this soon rises to 100–200 ml ten times a day by the tenth day of life.
9 The ability to control voiding of urine depends on a complete and functioning renal system, maturation of the nervous supply, opportunity/support given to the child to void and cultural expectations.
10 When the bladder fills it distends the trigone stretch receptors, and these in turn send impulses to the sacral area of the spine via the autonomic nervous system. Motor impulses from the spinal cord via the autonomic nervous system initiate relaxation of the internal sphincter and contraction of the detrusor muscle, leading to urine being consciously expelled.
11 A child's bladder capacity is estimated by age; age in years × 30 plus 30 = ml capacity. Thus, for a six-year-old child bladder capacity would be 210 ml and the child would be expected to visit the toilet around six to seven times a day.

12 The diagnosis of nocturnal enuresis is made when the involuntary passage of urine, during sleep, occurs in a child aged five years or more, in the absence of any congenital or acquired defects of the nervous system.
13 Deep sleep, food sensitivity such as citrus fruits, those who produce more urine than average, those who have small functional bladders (they normally pee more often than their peers), and those who are prone to constipation and thus their bladder expansion is restricted.
14 Skin turgor, respiratory pattern and the time blood takes to refill the nail bed, together with dry mucous membranes, sunken eyes and poor overall appearance plus the lack of tear production when assessing young children between one and thirty-six months and palpating for a sunken anterior fontanelle.
15 Isotonic dehydration is when water and electrolytes (especially sodium salt) are lost in equal amounts.
16 The best way to introduce water back into the body is through giving oral fluids. The solution recommended by the WHO contains sodium, potassium, chloride, base, glucose and water. Glucose is the preferred sugar because it facilitates the transport of sodium across the bowel wall.
17 As the extracellular sodium dilutes, water moves into the cells and cerebral and pulmonary oedema develops.
18 Eat bananas, dates and raisins.
19 One way is to attach a collecting plastic bag over the urethral opening – easier in boys than girls – or place a collection pad/cotton ball in the nappy/pants/knickers. The parent/carer can also be requested to catch a clean sample from a toddler who is left without a nappy until they void.
20 Appearance should be straw coloured; if concentrated it will be a dark orange, and if diluted a pale lemon colour. Red urine may reflect the diet of the previous day, for example beetroot. Jaundiced babies will have dark orange/brown urine due to the excretion of bile salts which should be excreted through the gut. Pink deposits from small babies are urates, not blood.

7 The digestive system

1 mouth
2 teeth
3 oesophagus
4 stomach
5 duodenum
6 ileum

7 caecum
8 colon
9 anus
10 smooth (muscle)
11 acid
12 peristalsis
13 chemical
14 mechanical

8 The reproductive system

A – androgens
B – breast
C – chromosome
D – deferens
E – endometrium
F – Fallopian tube
G – gene
H – hormone
I – inguinal
J – juvenile
K – kissing
L – Leidig cells
M – menarche
N – negative feedback
O – ovary
P – puberty

9 The immune system

1 Resistance to infection depends on general body defence mechanisms, innate genetic inheritance and an acquired passive or active resistance.
2 Intact skin and mucosa surfaces.
3 Injury due to infection, mechanical damage, ischemia (lack of oxygen supply), lack of nutrients, immune defects such as those children who are given cancer therapy, chemical agents, temperature extremes such as high fever or frost bite, and radiation such as sunburn.
4 The lymphoid type cells differentiate to T cells via the thymus gland responsible for virus attack and B cells via the liver and bone marrow itself responsible for bacterial attack.

5 Active immunity follows exposure and stimulation of the immune response to any infection, such as the common cold and chickenpox, or by immunisation against hepatitis, measles, mumps and rubella (MMR).

6 IgE is the immunoglobulin involved in allergic, anaphylactic and atopic reactions. The allergic individual responds to antigen invasion by combining the allergen with IgE rather than IgG, thus it is not phagocytosed. The IgE/antigen complex instead then stimulates mast cells in the tissues to produce histamine. Allergens such as pollen, certain foods, drugs, dust, insect venom and moulds.

7 It is IgG that is transported across the placenta to the greatest extent.

8 Rhesus iso-immunisation occurs when the foetus red cells carry rhesus positive antigen and the mother is rhesus negative. As foetal red cells can always enter the blood of the mother, she develops immunoglobulins against them of the IgM then IgG class.

9 The thymus is vital for the maturation of the T lymphocyte.

10 Differentiation of primitive lymphocytes, which have migrated from the bone marrow, into immuno-competent T cells.

11 It assists in maintaining the blood volume by collecting fluid, wastes and white blood cells that are in excess in the interstitial spaces.

12 Its vessels have 'blind' endings that open as tissue pressure builds up – a tissue pump.

13 In 'acute' stress, the cortex of the brain perceives a threatening situation and activates the autonomic nervous system sympathetic branch via the hypothalamus to release adrenaline and noradrenaline from the chromaffin cells in the adrenal medulla.

14 If the stressful situation continues, the hypothalamus activates a second system which affects the pituitary gland and its release of prolactin, growth hormone, endorphins and adrenocorticotropic hormone (ACTH), which stimulate the adrenal cortex to secrete cortisol.

15 Cortisol increases gastric acid secretion.

16 'The ability to bounce back' in the face of adversity; to know how and where and from whom to get support when problems arise.

17 Be a good role model, have a trusting and caring relationship with the young people, give them a sense of mastery over the tasks they are asked to perform, instil self confidence, help them to manage their feelings, respond to feelings of others and develop a sense of humour.

18 Live but weakened (attenuated) pathogenic micro-organisms stimulate the body to recognise a foreign (antigen) protein and produce antibodies to destroy it. The memory created protects the child from future invasion of the particular pathogen. MMR vaccine can induce a mild form of measles within ten days of vaccination and/or a general inflammatory response.

19 Toxoids, such as those from tetanus and diphtheria, are the modified bacterial toxins that have been made non-toxic, but which retain the ability to stimulate the formation of antibodies.
20 Some viruses are cultured for vaccines in egg tissue with antibiotics that suppress bacterial contamination. Some children may be hypersensitive and produce an allergic response to these foreign proteins, and release histamine into the tissues.

10 Body and mind

1 amygdale
2 behaviour
3 thinking
4 emotional
5 social
6 hippocampus
7 attention
8 ADHD
9 perception
10 infant
11 motivation
12 limbic
13 moral
14 hypothalamus
15 cognitive
16 memory
17 parent
18 ethnic
19 culture

References

1 Child physical needs

Barker, J. and Hodes, D. (2004) *The Child in Mind: A Child Protection Handbook*, London: Routledge.

Bee, H. and Boyd, D. (2007) *The Developing Child* (11th edition), Boston, MA: Pearson.

Bellaby, P. (2003) 'Communication and miscommunication of risk: understanding UK parents' attitudes to combined MMR vaccination', *BMJ*, 327 (7417): 725–772.

Boreham, C. and Riddock, C. (2001) 'The physical activity, fitness and health of children', *Journal of Sports Sciences*, 19(12): 915–929.

Bowlby, J. (2000) *The Making and Breaking of Affectionate Bonds*, London: Routledge.

Carnidge, D.R., Wood, R.J. and Bateman, D.N. (2003) 'The epidemiology of self-poisoning in the UK', *BJ Clinical Pharmacology*, 56(6) 613–619.

Cawson, D., Wattam, C., Brooker, S. and Kelly, G. (2000) *Child Maltreatment in the UK: A Study of the Prevalence of Abuse and Neglect*, available online at www.nspcc.org.uk/inform, accessed July 2007.

Chan, J. (1995) 'Dietary beliefs of Chinese patients', *Nursing Standard*, 9(27): 30–34.

Chief Medical Officer (2006) *Planned Changes to the Routine Childhood Immunisation Programme: Letter to Professionals*, 8 February, London: The Stationery Office.

Coombes, R. (2007) 'Life saving treatment or giant experiment', *BMJ*, 334 (7596): 721–723.

Corby, B. (2006) *Child Abuse: Towards a Knowledge Base* (3rd edition), Maidenhead: Oxford University Press.

Costain, L. (2007) 'Eating well – children and food', available online at www.bbc.co.uk/health, accessed 27 April 2007.

Cox, H. (2006) 'Food allergy in infants', *Community Practitioner*, 79(12): 406–407.

Department for Education and Employment (1999) *National Healthy School Standard: Getting Started – A Guide for Schools*, London: DFEE.

Department for Education and Skills (2006) *Working Together to Safeguard Children: Every Child Matters, Change for Children*, London: The Stationery Office.

Department of Health (1999) *Saving Lives: Our Healthier Nation*, London: The Stationery Office.

Department of Health (2003) *The Victoria Climbe Inquiry: Report of the Inquiry by Lord Laming*, London: The Stationery Office.

Diggle, L. (2006) 'Childhood immunisation', *Community Practitioner*, 79(7): 231–232.

Furber, C. and Thomson, A. (2006) 'Breaking the rules in baby feeding practice in the UK: deviance and good practice', *Midwifery*, 22(4): 365–376.

Glasper, A., McEwing, G. and Richardson, J. (2007) *Oxford Handbook of Children's and Young People's Nursing*, Oxford: Oxford University Press.

Gross, R.D. (2005) *Psychology: The Science of Mind and Behaviour* (5th edition), London: Hodder Arnold.

Haines, L., Wan, K., Lunn, R., Barrett, T. and Shield, J. (2007) *Diabetes Care*, American Diabetic Association, 30: 1097–1101. Available online at www.healthline.com, accessed July 2007.

Hall, D. and Elliman, D. (2003) *Health for all Children* (4th edition), Oxford: Oxford University Press.

Holden, C. and MacDonald, A. (2000) *Nutrition and Child Health*, London: Bailliere.

Jones, C.A., Holloway, J.A. and Warner, J. (2002) 'Foetal immune responsiveness and routes of allergic sensitization', *Paediatric Allergy Immunology*, 13(15): s19–s22.

Jose, N. (2005) 'Child poverty: is it child abuse', *Paediatric Nursing*, 17(8): 20–23.

Kmietowicz, Z. (2006) 'Children worldwide can grow to the same height', *BMJ*, 332: 1052 (6 May).

London, M., Ladewig, P., Ball, J. and Bindler, R. (2006) *Maternal and Child Nursing Care* (2nd edition), London: Prentice Hall.

McCance, K.L. and Heuther, S.E. (2006) *Pathophysiology: The Biological Basis for Disease in Adults and Children* (5th edition), St Louis, MO: Elsevier.

MacNair, T. (2007) 'Eating well – a balanced diet'. Available online at www.bbc.co.uk/health, accessed 27 April 2007.

McQuaid, L., Huband, S. and Esther, M.P. (eds) (1996) *Children's Nursing*, Edinburgh: Churchill Livingstone.

Magnusson, J. (2005) 'Childhood obesity: prevention, treatment and recommendations for health', *Community Practitioner*, 784: 147–149.

Marieb, E. and Hoehn, K. (2007) *Human Anatomy and Physiology* (7th edition), San Francisco, CA: Pearson.

Peate, I. and Whiting, L. (2006) *Caring for Children*, London: Wiley.

Pender, N.J., Murdaugh, C.C. and Parsons, M.A. (2002) *Health Promotion in Nursing Practice* (4th edition), Upper Saddle River, NJ: Prentice Hall.

Polnay, L. (2002) *Community Paediatrics* (3rd edition), Edinburgh: Livingstone.

Reilly, J., Armstrong, J., Dorosty, A., Emmett, P., Ness, A. *et al.* (2005) 'Early life risk factors for obesity in children', *BMJ* 330 (7504): 1357.

Roberts, I., DiGuiseppi, C. and Ward, H. (1998) 'Childhood injuries: extent of the problem, epidemilogical trends, and costs', *Injury Prevention*, 4: s10–s16.

Robinson, S. (2006) *Healthy Eating in Primary Schools*, London: Sage.

Rudolf, M. and Leucene, M. (1999) *Pediatrics and Child Health*, London: Blackwell Science.

Samad, A. (2006) 'Differences in risk factors for partial and no immunisation in the first year of life', *BMJ*, 332 (7553): 1312–1313.

Takano,T. and Nakamura, K. (2001) 'An analysis of health levels and various indicators of urban environment', *Journal of Epidemiology Community Health*, 55(4): 263–270.

Taylor, L. Gallagher, M. and McCullough, M. (2004) 'The role of parental influence and additional factors in the determination of food choices for pre-school children', *International Journal of Consumer Studies*, 28(4): 337–341.

Thibodeau, G.A. and Patton, K.T. (2007) *Anatomy and Physiology* (18th edition), London: Mosby.

Trigge, E. and Mohammed, T. (2006) *Practices in Children's Nursing* (2nd edition), London: Elsevier.

Turner, A. (2002) *Occupational Therapy and Physical Dysfunction: Principles, Skills and Practice* (5th edition), Edinburgh: Churchill Livingstone.

Twinn, S., Roberts, B. and Andrews, S. (1998) *Community Health Care Nursing*, Oxford: Butterworth.

UNICEF (2007) *Report Card 7 – Poverty in Perspective: An Overview of Child Well-being in Rich Countries*, Florence: Innocenti Research Centre. Available online at www.news.bbc.co.uk/1/hi/uk/6359363.stm, accessed 3 March 2007.

Venter, C. (2006) 'Food hypersensitivity amongst children on the Isle of Wight: an in-depth dietry investigation', unpublished Ph.D. thesis, University of Southampton.

Viner, R. and Booy, R. (2005) 'ABC of adolescence: epidemiology of health and illness', *BMJ*, 330 (7488): 411–414.

Werner, E. and Smith, R. (2001) *Journeys from Childhood to Midlife: Risk, Resilience and Recovery*, Ithaca, NY: Cornell University Press.

Wilkinson, S. and Walker, A. (2007) 'Healthy start: improving maternal, infant and child health', *Nursing Standard*, 21(20): 48–55.

Wong, D., Hockenberry, M.J., Wilson, D., Winkelstein, M.L. and Kline, N.E. (2003) *Nursing Care of Infants and Children* (6th edition), St Louis, MO: Mosby.

www.eatwell.gov.uk/ages
www.everychildmatters.gov.uk/socialcare/safeguarding
www.healthline.com
www.immunisation.nhs.uk
www.who.int/childgrowth/en/

2 The skeletal system

Bailey, D.A. and Martin, A.D. (1994) 'Physical activity and skeletal health in adolescents', *Pediatric Exercise Science*, 6(4): 330–347.

Branca, F. (1999) 'Physical activity, diet and skeletal health', *Public Health Nutrition*, 2(3a): 391–396.

Geissler, C. and Powers, H. (2005) *Human Nutrition* (11th edition), Edinburgh: Elsevier.

Jenkins, G.W., Kemnitz, C.P. and Tortora, G.J. (2007) *Anatomy and Physiology*, Hoboken, NJ: Wiley and Sons.

Kahn, S.A., Pace, J.E. and Cox, M. (1994) 'Osteoporosis and genetic influence: a three generation study', *Postgraduate Medical Journal*, 829(70): 798–800.

Mallan, K., Metcalf, B.S., Kirkby, I., Voss, L. and Wilkin, T. (2003) 'Contribution of timetabled physical education to total physical activity in primary school children: cross sectional study', *BMJ*, 327(7415): 592–593.

May, P., Ashford, E. and Bottle, G. (2006) *Sound Beginnings; Learning and Development*, London: David Fulton Publishers.

Morris, F.L., Naughton, G.A., Gibbs, J.L., Carlson, J.S. and Waik, J.B. (1997) 'Prospective ten month exercise intervention in premenarcheal girls', *Journal of Bone Mineral Research*, 12: 1453–1463.

Neill, S. and Knowles, H. (eds) (2004) *The Biology of Child Health: A Reader in Development and Assessment*, Basingstoke: Palgrave Macmillan.

Patel, S., Duche, P. and Williamson, C.A. (2006) 'Muscle fatigue during high intensity exercise in children', *Sports Medicine*, 36(12): 1031–1065.

Pellegrini, A.D. and Smith, P.K. (1998) 'Physical activity play: the nature and function of a neglected aspect of play', *Child Development*, 69(3): 577–598.

Rodriguez, G.V. (2006) 'How does exercise affect bone development during growth?', *Sports Medicine*, 36(7): 561–569.

Siranda, J. and Pate, R. (2001) 'Physical activity assessment in children and adolescents', *Sports Medicine*, 31(6): 439–454.

Tanner, J.M. (1989) *Foetus into Man* (2nd edition), Ware: Castlemead.

Thibodeau, G.A. and Patton, K.T. (2007) *Anatomy and Physiology* (18th edition), St. Louis, MO: Mosby.

Voss, L.D., Mulligan, J. and Betts, P.R. (1998) 'Short stature at school entry: an index of social deprivation? Wessex Growth Study', *Child Care, Health and Development*, 24(2): 145–156.
Watts, K., Jones, T., Davis, E. and Green, D. (2005) 'Exercise training in obese children and adolescents', *Sports Medicine*, 35(5): 375–392.
Wood, E. and Attfield, J. (2006) *Play, Learning and the Early Childhood Curriculum* (2nd edition), London: Sage.

www.fph.org.uk

3 The nervous system

Bear, M., Connors, B. and Paradiso, M. (2007) *Neuroscience, Exploring the Brain* (3rd edition), London: Lippincott, Williams and Wilkins.
Bee, H. and Boyd, D. (2007) *The Developing Child* (11th edition), Boston, MA: Pearson.
Carlson, N. (2001) *Physiology of Behaviour* (7th edition), Boston, MA: Allyn and Bacon, Pearson Educational Co.
Casey, G. (2000) 'Fever management', *Paediatric Nursing*, 12(3): 38–42.
Edwards, S. (1998) 'High temperature', *Professional Nurse*, 13(8): 521–526.
Glasper, A., McEwing, G. and Richardson, J. (eds) (2007) *Oxford Handbook of Children's and Young People's Nursing*, Oxford: Oxford University Press.
Harris, M. and Butterworth, G. (2002) *Developmental Psychology*, London: Psychology Press.
Laberge, L., Petit, D., Simard, C., Vitaro, F., Tremblay, R. and Montplaisir, J. (2001) 'Development of sleep patterns in early adolescence', *Journal of Sleep Research*, 10(1): 59–67.
Levin, R. and Neilson, T. (2007) 'Disturbed dreaming, post-traumatic stress disorder and affective distress: a review and neurocognitive model', *Psychological Bulletin*, 133(3): 482–528.
London, M., Ladewig, P., Ball, J. and Bindler, R. (2006) *Maternal and Child Nursing Care* (2nd edition), Upper Saddle River, NJ: Prentice Hall.
Marieb, E. and Hoehn, K. (2007) *Human Anatomy and Physiology* (7th edition), San Francisco, CA: Pearson.
McNeilly, P. (2004) 'Complementary therapies for children: aromatherapy', *Paediatric Nursing*, 16(7): 28–30.
Moyse, K. (2005) 'Baby massage and baby play: promoting touch and stimulation in early childhood', *Paediatric Nursing*, 17(5): 30–32.
Sadeh, A. (2004) 'A brief screening questionnaire for infant sleep problems: validation and findings for an internet sample', *Pediatrics*, 113(6): 570–577.
Sadeh, A., Gruber R. and Raviv, A. (2002) 'Sleep, neurobehavioural functioning and behaviour problems in school aged children', *Child Development*, 73(2): 405–417.

www.nice.org.uk

4 The cardiovascular system

Armstrong, N. (2006) *Paediatric Exercise Science and Medicine*, Edinburgh: Churchill Livingstone.
Baker, P. (ed.) (2006) *Obstetrics by Ten Teachers* (18th edition), London: Hodder.
Boreham, C., Twisk, J., Murray, L., Savage, M., Strain, J. and Cran, G. (2001) 'Fitness, fatness and coronary heart disease risk in adolescents: the Northern Ireland Young Hearts project', *Medicine and Science in Sports and Exercise*, 33(2): 270–274.

Halazinski, M. (1992) *Nursing Care of the Critically Ill Child*, St Louis, MO: Mosby.

Hippisley-Cox, J., Coupland, C., Vinogradora, Y., Robson, J., May, M. and Brindle, P. (2007) 'Derivation and validation of QRISK: a new CVD risk score for the United Kingdom, prospective open cohort study', *BMJ*, 335(7611): 136.

Jackson, L., Thalange, N. and Cole, T. (2006) 'Blood pressure centiles for Great Britain', *Archives of Diseases in Children*, 92(4): 298–303.

Lissauer, T. and Clayden, G. (2004) *Illustrated Textbook of Paediatrics* (2nd edition), London: Mosby.

McCance, K.L. and Heuther, S.E. (2006) *Pathophysiology: The Biological Basis for Disease in Adults and Children* (5th edition), St Louis, MO: Elsevier.

McLeod, K.A. (2003) 'Syncope in childhood', *Archives of Disease in Childhood*, 88(4): 350–353.

Marieb, E. and Hoehn, K. (2007) *Anatomy and Physiology* (7th edition), San Francisco, CA: Pearson.

Moore, K. (2003) *Before We Are Born: Essentials of Embryology and Birth Defects*, Philadelphia, PA: Saunders.

Summer, K. (2007) 'Evidence-based practice: non-invasive blood pressure measurement in children', *Journal of Children's and Young People's Nursing*, 1(2): 59–63.

Thureen, P.J., Deacon, J., Hernandez, J.A. and Hall, D. (2004) *Assessment and Care of the Well Newborn* (2nd edition), London: W.B. Saunders.

Wallis, L.A. and Maconochie, I. (2006) 'Age-related reference ranges of respiratory and heart rate for children in South Africa', *Archives of Diseases in Children*, 91(4): 330–333.

Wallis, L.A., Healey, M., Undy, M.B. and Maconochie, I. (2005) 'Age-related reference ranges for respiration rate and heart rate for 4 to 16 years', *Archives of Diseases in Children*, 90(11): 1117–1121.

www.aap.org/topics.html, accessed 2 February 2008
www.nspku.org
www.screening.nhs.uk
www.newbornscreening.bloodspot.org.uk

5 The respiratory system

Arets, B. (2007) 'Healthy children with smoking parents – are they really healthy?', paper presented at the American Thoracic Society 2007 International Conference, 20 May 2007 (Session A105, Abstract # 309). Available online at www.sciencedaily.com, accessed July 2007.

Armstrong, N. (ed.) (2007) *Paediatric Exercise Physiology*, London: Elsevier.

Aylott, M. (2006) 'The neonatal energy triangle. Part 2: Thermoregulatory and respiratory adaptation', *Paediatric Nursing*, 18(7): 38–42.

Baker, P. (ed.) (2006) *Obstetrics by Ten Teachers* (18th edition), London: Hodder.

Booker, R. (2007) 'Peak expiratory flow measurement', *Nursing Standard*, 21(39): 42–43.

Boran, P., Tokuc, G., Pisgin, B., Oktem, S., Yegin, Z. and Bostan, O. (2007) 'Impact of obesity on ventilatory function', *Journal de Pediatria*, 83(2): 171–176.

Chandler, T. (2000) 'Oxygen saturation monitoring', *Paediatric Nursing*, 12(8): 37–42.

Gauderman, W.J., Vora, H., McConnell, R., Berhane, K., Gilliland, F., *et al.* (2007) 'Effect of exposure to traffic on lung development from 10–18 years of age: a cohort study', *The Lancet*, 369(9561): 570–577.

Marieb, E. and Hoehn, K. (2007) *Anatomy and Physiology* (7th edition), San Francisco, CA: Pearson.

Tantucci, C., Dugnet, A., Giampiccolo, P., Similowski, T., Zelter, M. and Devenne, J. (2002) 'The best peak expiratory flow is flow-limited and effort-independent in normal subjects', *American Journal of Respiratory and Critical Care Medicine*, 165: 1304–1308.

Thibodeau, G. and Patton, K. (2007) *Anatomy Physiology* (18th edition), London: Mosby.
Uliel, S., Tauman, R., Greenfield, M. and Sivan, Y. (2004) 'Normal polysommographic respiratory values in children and adolescents', *Chest*, 125(3): 872–878.
Wallis, L.A., Healy, M., Undy, M.B. and Maconochie, I. (2005) 'Age-related reference ranges for respiration rate and heart rate for 4 to 16 years', *Archives of Diseases in Children*, 90(11): 1117–1121.

www.blobs.org/science/anatomy
www.clinicalevidence.com
www.entnet.org
www.fsid.org.uk
www.nhsdirect.nhs.uk, accessed July 2007
www.resus.org.uk

6 The renal system

Chamley, C., Carson, P., Randell, D. and Sandwell, M. (2005) *Developmental Anatomy and Physiology of Children*, Edinburgh: Churchill Livingstone.
Freidman, J., Goldman, R., Srivastava, R. and Parkin, C. (2004) 'Development of a clinical dehydration scale for use in children between 1 and 36 months of age', *Journal of Pediatrics*, 145(2): 201–207.
Glasper, E., McEwing, G. and Richardson, J. (eds) (2007) *Oxford Handbook of Children's and Young People's Nursing*, Oxford: Oxford University Press.
Kamperis, K. and Djurhuus, J. (2006) 'For some bed wetters, sodium' prostaglandin may be key to successful treatment'. Available online at www.medicalnewstoday.com/articles/57960php, accessed July 2007.
Kaushik, A., Mullee, M., Bryant, T. and Hill, C. (2007) 'A study of the association between children's access to drinking water in primary schools and their fluid intake; can water be "cool" at school?', *Child Care, Health and Development*, 33(4): 409–415.
London, M., Ladewig, P., Ball, J. and Bindler, R. (2007) *Maternal and Child Nursing Care* (2nd edition), Upper Saddle River, NJ: Pearson Education.
Marieb, E. and Hoehn, K. (2007) *Anatomy and Physiology* (7th edition), San Francisco, CA: Pearson.
McCance, K.L. and Heuther, S.E. (2006) *Pathophysiology: The Biological Basis for Disease in Adults and Children* (5th edition), St Louis, MO: Elsevier.
Mercer, R. 'Bed wetting facts'. Available online at www.bedwettingstore.com, accessed December 2007.
Steiner, M.J., DeWalt, D.A. and Byerley, J.S. (2004) 'Review: capillary refill time, abnormal skin turgor, and abnormal respiratory pattern are useful signs for detecting dehydration in children', *Journal of the American Medical Association*, 291(21): 2746–2754.
Van Hoek, K., Bael, A. and Lax, H. (2007) 'Circadian variation of voided volume in normal school-age children', *European Journal of Pediatrics*, 166(6): 579–584.

www.intesivecaring.com, accessed July 2007
www.medicalnewstonight.com, accessed July 2007
www.nlm.nih.gov/medlineplus/ency/article002220, accessed July 2007

7 The digestive system

Baker, P. (2005) 'Diet and behaviour'. Available online at http://news.bbc.co.uk, accessed 14 October 2005.

Catto-Smith, A. (2005) 'Constipation and toileting issues in children', *The Medical Journal of Australia*, 182(5): 242–246.
Cole, T., Flegal, K., Nicolls, D. and Jackson, A. (2007) 'Body mass index cut offs to define thinness in children and adolescents: international survey', *BMJ*, 335 (7612): 166–167.
Geissler, C. and Powers, H. (2005) *Human Nutrition* (11th edition), Edinburgh: Churchill Livingstone.
Goyal, R. and Mashimo, H. (2006) 'Physiology of oral, pharangeal and oesophageal motility'. Available online at www.nature.com/gimo/contents/pt1/full/giom1.html, accessed 6 February 2008.
Levine, R., Nugent, Z., Rudolf, M. and Sahota, P. (2007) 'Dietry patterns, tooth brushing habits and caries experience of school children in West Yorkshire, England', *Community Dental Health*, 24(2): 82–87.
Marieb, E. and Hoehn, K. (2007) *Anatomy and Physiology* (7th edition), San Francisco, CA: Pearson.
Quiros-Tejeira, R. (2007) 'Risk for non-alcoholic fatty liver disease in Hispanic youth with BMI above 95centile', *Journal of Gastroenterology and Nutrition*, 44(2): 228–236.

www.aboutkidshealth.ca
www.babycentre.co.uk, accessed August 2007
www.babyledweaning.com
www.keepkidshealthy.com, accessed 9 September 2007
www.organix.com
www.teething-babies.co.uk
www.weightlossresources.co.uk
www.who.com

8 The reproductive system

Bunc, V. and Dlouha, R. (2000) 'Estimation of body composition by multifrequency bioimpedance measurement, in vivo Body Composition Studies', *Annals New York Academy Sciences*, 904(1): 203–207.
McCance, K.L. and Heuther, S.E. (2006) *Pathophysiology: The Biological Basis for Disease in Adults and Children* (5th edition), St Louis, MO: Elsevier.
Marieb, E. and Hoehn, K. (2007) *Anatomy and Physiology* (7th edition), San Francisco, CA: Pearson.
Simonsen, T., Aarbakke, J., Kay, I., Coleman, I., Sinnott, P. and Lysaa, R. (2006) *Illustrated Pharmacology for Nurses*, London: Hodder Arnold.
Tripp, J. and Viner, R. (2005) 'Sexual health, contraception and teenage pregnancy', *BMJ*, 330(7491): 590–593.
Viner, R. and Barker, M. (2005) 'Young people's health; the need for action', *BMJ*, 330(7496): 901–903.
Wang, T., Morioka, I., Gowa, Y., Igarashi, Y., Miyai, N., *et al.* (2004) 'Serum leptin levels in healthy adolescents: effects of gender and growth', *Environmental Health and Preventive Medicine*, 9(2): 41–46.

http://womenshealth.about.com, accessed August 2007
www.alspac.bristol.ac.uk, accessed 14 August 2007
www.fda.gov, accessed August 2007
www.news.bbc.co.uk, accessed 14 August 2007
www.kidshealth.org, accessed August 2007
www.patient.co.uk, accessed August 2007
www.thechildrenshospital.org, accessed August 2007

9 The immune system

Bee, H. and Boyd, D. (2007) *The Developing Child* (11th edition), Boston, MA: Pearson.
Marieb, E. and Hoehn, K. (2007) *Anatomy and Physiology* (7th edition), San Francisco, CA: Pearson.
McCance, K.L. and Heuther, S.E. (2006) *Pathophysiology: The Biological Basis for Disease in Adults and Children* (5th edition), St Louis, MO: Elsevier.
Montgomery, S.M., Ehlin, A. and Sacker, A. (2006) 'Breast feeding and resilience against psychosocial stress', *Archives of Diseases in Children*, 91(12): 990–994.
Playfair, J.H.L. and Chain, B.M. (2001) *Immunology at a Glance* (7th edition), Oxford: Blackwell Science.
Scavelli, C., Weber, E., Aglianò, M., Cirulli, T., Nico, B. *et al.* (2004) 'Lymphatics at the crossroads of angiogenesis and lymphangiogenesis', *Journal of Anatomy*, 204(6): 433–449.
Stevenson, O. (2007) *Neglected Children and their Families* (2nd edition), Oxford: Blackwell Publishing.

http://hcd2.bupa.co.uk
www.allergyuk.org
www.direct.gov.uk
www.healthpromotingschools.co.uk
www.immunization.nhs.uk
www.patient.co.uk
www.scotland.gov.uk

10 Body and mind

Bee, H. and Boyd, D. (2007) *The Developing Child* (11th edition), Boston, MA: Pearson.
Bowlby, J. (1951) *Maternal Care and Mental Health*, Geneva: WHO.
Dosani, S. (2006) 'Prevention of psychosocial problems in adolescence', *BMJ*, 333(7566): 460.
Evans, G. (2006) 'Child development and the physical environment', *Psychology Annual Reviews*, 57: 423–451.
Gross, R. (2005) *Psychology: The Science of Mind and Behaviour* (5th edition), London: Hodder Arnold.
Marieb, E. and Hoehn, K. (2007) *Anatomy and Physiology* (7th edition), San Francisco, CA: Pearson.
Maslow, A. (1954) *Motivation and Personality*, New York: Harper.
Meadows, S. (1996) *Parenting Behaviour and Children's Cognitive Behaviour*, Hove: Psychology Press.
Slee, P. and Shute, R. (2003) *Child Development: Thinking about Theories*, London: Hodder Arnold.
Vorria, P., Papaligoura, Z., Sarafidon, J., Kipakaki, M., Dunn, J., *et al.* (2006) 'The development of adopted children after institutional care: a follow-up study', *Journal of Child Psychology and Psychiatry*, 47(12): 1246–1253.

Index